Praise for

FAMILY FUN AND FITNESS

Family Fun and Fitness is a book that every parent concerned about their child's health (and their own health) must have. Childhood obesity has reached epidemic proportions, but the truth is that children's habits are formed from their parent's example. This book provides parents with easy-to-use, effective information and tips that will permanently benefit the *whole* family's health. If you love your children . . . and who doesn't . . . *Family Fun and Fitness* is a *must* have.

—JORGE E. RODRIGUEZ, M.D., INTERNIST, ORANGE COAST MEDICAL GROUP,
AND MEDICAL CONSULTANT ON ABC'S *THE VIEW*

Preventive medicine effectively starts at birth. As a physician who has practiced internal medicine and cardiology for more than fifty years, I have spent the greater part of this time treating the results of disease that could have been prevented. *Family Fun and Fitness* is an excellent book that shows the way, from the very beginning, to achieve good health for your family.

—EUGENE B. LEVIN, M.D., F.A.C.P., INTERNIST AND CARDIOLOGIST,
PACIFIC CREST MEDICAL GROUP, LAGUNA BEACH, CA

Family Fun and Fitness successfully captures the importance of a healthy family lifestyle. This book gives inventive suggestions, motivating ideas, and strong healthy direction that parents need for their children. I highly recommend *Family Fun and Fitness* to all families.

—EDWARD L. SMITH, D.O., FAMILY PRACTITIONER, PERSONAL
AND FAMILY HEALTHCARE, LAGUNA NIGUEL, CA

Family Fun and Fitness is a must for parents who want to optimize the health of their children in our increasingly sedentary and fast-food-filled world. This book contains the essentials parents need to create a home environment conducive to a healthy family lifestyle. We all know that leading by example is the best way to teach our children, and if you follow these recommendations the whole family will be healthier because of it.

—ROBERT KESSLER, M.D., F.A.C.S., AESTHETIC SURGEON AND CONSULTANT ON ABC'S EXTREME MAKEOVER

FAMILY FUN AND FITNESS

Getting Healthy and Staying Healthy—Together

KNUTE KEELING

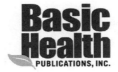

Basic Health
PUBLICATIONS, INC.

The information contained in this book is based upon the research and personal and professional experiences of the author. It is not intended as a substitute for consulting with your physician or other healthcare provider. Any attempt to diagnose and treat an illness should be done under the direction of a healthcare professional.

The publisher does not advocate the use of any particular healthcare protocol but believes the information in this book should be available to the public. The publisher and author are not responsible for any adverse effects or consequences resulting from the use of the suggestions, preparations, or procedures discussed in this book. Should the reader have any questions concerning the appropriateness of any procedures or preparation mentioned, the author and the publisher strongly suggest consulting a professional healthcare advisor.

Basic Health Publications, Inc.
28812 Top of the World Drive
Laguna Beach, CA 92651
949-715-7327 • www.basichealthpub.com

Library of Congress Cataloging-in-Publication Data

Keeling, Knute
    Family fun and fitness : getting healthy and staying healthy-together /
Knute Keeling.
        p. cm.
    Includes bibliographical references and index.
    ISBN 978-1-59120-255-4
    1. Children—Health and hygiene—Popular works. 2. Physical fitness
for children—Popular works. I. Title.
    RJ61.K257   2009
    613'.0432—dc22

                                                            2009026735

Editor: Cheryl Hirsch
Typesetting/Graphic design: Gary A. Rosenberg
Cover design: Mike Stromberg

Printed in the United States of America

10   9   8   7   6   5   4   3   2   1

Contents

Dedicated to my best friend and wife, Nikki,
and our beautiful daughters, Cameron and Kianna,
who have made my life go from black and white to color.

The fun and spirit of our family
inspired the idea and vision for this book.

Acknowledgments

I am grateful to many family and friends who have formed my foundation as a family man. I would like to first acknowledge Melissa Lynn Block for her amazing writing skills and for her ability to take all this information and put it together for this book. I would like to also acknowledge Tracey Bouknight for her photography and wonderful artistic ideas. I would like to give special thanks to Norman Goldfind at Basic Health Publications for listening to my idea and for believing in this important material.

I would like to give thanks in addition to Dr. Bruce Connell, Dennis Camene, and Jon Madison for their friendship, advice, and amazing support of my family.

I would like to also acknowledge my parents for all their adventurous camping trips that involved fishing, swimming, and nature walks. These healthy childhood experiences helped instill in me a sense of the importance of family fitness, which is what this book is all about.

I would like to also thank my best man, Colin Cashin, and his beautiful wife, Michelle, along with their incredible kids. This "studly" family is the healthiest, most active family I know. Thank you Cashins for all the great Thanksgiving Day dinners, and thanks, Colin, for the intense rock climbing at Joshua Tree National Park, the scuba diving in Catalina, and that crazy climb of Mount San Jacinto Peak.

Finally, I would like to acknowledge Margie and Joe Peeler of Oklahoma, who gave me a place to live while in school. Thanks for going to all my football games and for making me a special part of your family up to this very day! I will always be grateful to you for taking me in as a young man and for teaching me the family values that I continue to live by with my own family.

Introduction

You care deeply about the health of your children. You want them to be fit and happy and to do well in school and in life. Looking back, even from your present wiser, more seasoned vantage point, you know how hard it can be to be a kid . . . how irresistible it can be to indulge in less-than-healthful habits . . . and yet how much good health matters.

You're a good parent, a motivated parent, a parent who is willing to go the extra yard for the benefit of your family. If you weren't, you wouldn't have bothered to pick up this book. Of course, you want to give your children the best possible start. And you know that a major aspect of a great start in life includes being at a healthy weight and fitness level and eating healthfully. But you're up against some formidable adversaries:

- A huge variety of high-calorie, intensely sweet or salty, delicious, brightly colored, ingeniously packaged and advertised foods—some of which are served to your child when you aren't around. Even the best-intentioned parent who never gives his or her children these sorts of foods will be faced with a child who's hooked when he comes home wild-eyed from a party, face and hands sticky with sugar and artificial colorings, raving about the cake, and stuffing goodie-bag treats into his mouth.

- Some of the most engaging entertainment ever created—video games, computer games, computer-based socializing—all which involve (for the most part) sitting and staring at a screen.

Oversized portions of bad-for-your-kids foods are everywhere. They are rewarded with sweet treats at school and may be eating school lunch-

1

es that leave much to be desired in terms of nutrition. Sedentary leisure activities are taking over where playgrounds and neighborhood backyards once predominated. Schools and home life are conspiring to keep your kids from getting the physical activity they need. As a result, children are getting fatter and unhealthier with each passing year.

According to Trust for America's Health, an independent research group, one-third of America's children are overweight, and the percentage of American children who are heavy enough to be categorized as obese (what this means, exactly, you'll learn later in this book) has more than tripled since the 1970s.

Although your daughter might only be concerned about her weight because she wants to look like a stick-thin celebrity, you know that the problems with being heavy go well beyond this concern. Being obese is a health risk. Sure, you can be fit and eat healthy and be overweight—the research proves this. But for the most part, a person who is obese is not eating well or exercising regularly, and is at risk for a long laundry list of scary diseases, including type 2 diabetes and heart disease. A child who is obese is likely to start facing these health problems well before hitting late-middle age. Type 2 diabetes used to be called *adult-onset* diabetes because pediatricians almost never saw it in their patients. That has changed. For the first time in U.S. history, this current generation of kids is expected to have a lifespan shorter than the one before it.

This book contains all the tools you need to begin taking control of your family's health and doing all you can to ensure that your child gets the best possible start.

- In Chapter 1, "Kids in Crisis: The Big Picture of Children's Health," you'll learn more about the state of our health and the roadblocks in the way of moving into a more energized, fit way of life. You'll be invited to make a serious commitment to the fitness, good nutrition, and health of your whole family—and to set a better example with your own habits.

- In Chapter 2, "A Really Good Start: Pre-pregnancy, Prenatal, and Postpartum Nutrition and Fitness," you'll see how you can set the stage for optimal nutrition and fitness for your kids *before they are even born* and in the earliest months of their lives. This chapter will also help new moms to get back into a fitness and diet plan that will help shed pregnancy weight and begin to get them into the best shape of their lives after giving birth. As a parent myself of two beautiful little girls, I know that convenience and ease are crucial for new mothers, and so I've given you some ideas about how to work out and prepare healthful foods that I know can fit into the hectic schedule of a new mom.

- Chapter 3, "Fit Family Food Fundamentals," gives a broad, comprehensive overview of healthful eating for your whole family. You'll learn about fats, carbs, serving sizes, and tips and tricks to get kids to love eating foods that are good for them.

- Chapter 4, "Fit Family Food Plan," is a roadmap for parents who want to help their little ones get just the right start as they begin to make their own food choices. You'll learn how breastfeeding and holding and carrying your baby as much as possible in the early months of life play into this scenario. It will help you to find novel ways to sneak vegetables into your child, and to teach kids from a young age about which foods are nourishing for their bodies—and what that means.

- The next chapter, Chapter 5, "Fitness-Loving Kids: Fitness for School-Aged Children and Their Parents," includes my playground workout for busy moms, plus other workout plans and practical ideas for getting yourself *and* your kids excited about being fit and active.

- I'm especially excited to share with you the information in Chapter 6, "Fit Family, Smart Family, Happy Family," which is all about how an active, fit lifestyle and whole-food-rich, healthy diet promote optimal mental health, physical health, and achievement in school and at work.

- Finally, in Chapter 7, "Secrets of Fit, Energized Families," you'll get—straight from parents who have found ways to maintain a family fitness plan and a nutrition-packed diet—practical advice that will help you over and around any roadblocks you encounter as you strive to get your own family on track. In the back of the book, I'll supply recipes and other information that will help you further.

Think of me as your family's personal trainer. This is what I have done for the past twenty years in Laguna Beach, California. I've helped a lot of people meet their fitness and nutrition goals, and you're next.

Now, I know that this is going to be more difficult for some families than for others. Just as body weight, body fat distribution, and 'foodways' (cultural traditions that may include foods that are less than nutritious or high in calories) are dictated through genes and family traditions, so too is the urge to get enough exercise. The truth is that for some people, exercise will feel better than for others, and will be easier to stick with over time. Some people feel just fine without getting a workout five times a week, thanks very much.

Always remember, however, that you have to set the example for your kids if they're to eat healthfully and stay fit. Children can't change sedentary lifestyles, poor exercise habits, or eating habits on their own. They need direction, encouragement, and strong involvement from parents to be successful in moving toward better habits. The equation here is simple: *healthy, active parents equal healthy, active kids*. Even if it's hard, it's still the right thing to do. My client Kathleen Buchanan, a fit parent who has made exercise a priority in her life, puts it this way:

> From the age of seven, my four younger siblings and I swam competitively for the El Monte Aquatics AAU swim team. We worked out six days a week, with double-days on Saturday during the summer. While I was not always thrilled with this intense regimen, it instilled many valuable life lessons: team spirit, time management, and that chlorine can really mess with your hair color!
>
> Establishing a fitness regimen and healthy diet at an early age helped me realize the important role that exercise plays in relieving stress, enhancing sleep, and maintaining my healthy weight and outlook as an adult. Whether I participate in an aerobics class, take a run, power walk by myself, or work out with my inspiring trainer [thanks, Kathleen!], I have found that exercise is a critical component for me to maintain total body, mind, and spirit balance. The more active I am, the more energy I have to live my life to the fullest!

In this spirit, before you turn the page, hit the floor and give me twenty. Ten? Five? Or just take a short walk around the block, or climb your stairs a few times.

Let's get you and your family started on the road to lifelong fitness!

CHAPTER 1

Kids in Crisis:
The Big Picture
of Children's Health

The most important nutritional problem among children today is obesity . . . Obesity rates are rising rapidly among children and adolescents, especially those who are African American or Hispanic. The health consequences also are rising: 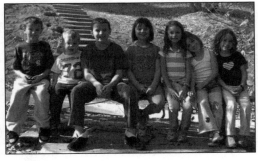 high levels of serum cholesterol, blood pressure, and "adult-onset" diabetes. This increase has occurred in response to complex societal, economic, demographic, and environmental changes that have reduced physical activity and promoted greater intake of foods high in calories but not necessarily high in nutrients.

—Marion Nestle, Ph.D., M.P.H.

One in three American children is overweight or obese. This isn't too big a surprise, considering that more than half of adults in the United States are overweight or obese as well.

The Centers for Disease Control and Prevention (CDC) has reported that the obesity rate in six- to eleven-year-olds has quintupled since 1970; for children between the ages of two and five and for teens, this rate has tripled. Ten percent of children between the ages of two and five, 15 percent of children between the ages of six and eleven, and 16 percent of children between the ages of twelve and nineteen are overweight or obese. In 1960, fewer than 5 percent of kids fit this description. And the figures for African-American and Hispanic children show double the rates of overweight and obesity. Teenagers in these ethnic groups are three times more likely to have weight issues.

Only 25 percent of adults with weight problems were overweight or obese as children. Weight gain in children isn't always to blame. But it's a factor, and a growing factor. You can do a lot for your children now to help them avoid tipping the scales too far in the future.

What does this mean, exactly? How did it happen? And what are the possible consequences? The probable consequences?

Before I get into that, I want to make something abundantly clear . . .

YOU DO NOT HAVE TO BE THIN TO BE FIT!

Yes, you read it right: Although being slim may be more likely to correspond with better health, this is only because obesity is what's known as a marker for an unhealthy lifestyle.

Unless you're blessed with the kind of genes that keep you thin no matter how much you eat, what you eat, or whether you exercise, you can't indulge in the average unhealthy lifestyle without it showing on your body in the form of excess weight. Children of parents who tend to put on excess pounds are more likely to do the same when they live that unhealthy lifestyle. But being a *fit* family does not have to involve being a *thin* family. Some people, even at their fittest, will fall into the category of "overweight" or even "obese."

In a Surgeon General's report published in the early 2000s, Steven Blair, M.D., wrote that "we need to stop hounding people about their weight and encourage them to eat healthful diets and exercise." This is true not only of adults, but also of children, who are so vulnerable to cultural messages about how they should look and to the hang-ups of their parents about their own bodies.

We need to emphasize with children from an early age that healthy bodies come in all shapes and sizes, and that this is not a bad thing, but a wonderful thing. We need to emphasize and embody the real truth about physical activity—that it gives us a great feeling of energy and exhilaration and an equally nice feeling of relaxed tiredness when we're done, and that it's a good time for family togetherness . . . and that we do it for those reasons, not to attain some idealized body dimensions. Eating a healthful diet feels great and gives us energy whether we're twig-thin or on the heavy side.

If you, the parent, see exercise and healthful eating as big drags on your enjoyment of life, and if you only follow fit habits because you want to look a certain way, you'll likely have two problems on your hands: first, you won't be able to stick with your program for any length of time; and second, you're going to send that message to your children.

So much emphasis is placed on weight loss and being slim, but the reality is that you can be extremely fit and healthy without having the body dimensions of a supermodel or sculpted celebrity! Although having a goal to look a certain way or fit into a certain size of clothing can be helpful in sticking with a program, in the end, your Fit Family Plan is about three things:

1. Time enjoying one another together as a family.

2. Children learning from parents during what I call *teachable moments* about how to feed their bodies, how to prepare the foods that are most nourishing, and how to get a great workout.

3. Finding ways to be active that are so much fun and so satisfying, energizing, and enriching that the activity becomes a part of the family's traditions and habits, not something done just to try to lose weight.

All this having been said: the sad truth is that the majority of people who are overweight or obese are also not living what I call the Fit Family Lifestyle. If you are reading this book, my guess is that you are looking to make a shift, and so part of my role here is to provide you with motivation. This requires that I share some potentially frightening information about the risks of overweight and obesity (when they are caused by poor diet and lack of physical activity). I offer this here because I know that sometimes people *need* to be shaken up a little to change their lives. My goal in this chapter is to motivate you to make the changes that will bring you and your family into your best possible health and to your ideal weight.

GETTING STARTED

The first step is to figure out where you are today by determining where you all fall in terms of body mass index (BMI). Refer to the inset below to calculate those numbers for each family member. Or, you can go online and search for "BMI Calculator" to find one of many sites where you enter height and weight and the site does the computation for you.

The Fit Family Plan is intended to guide you into a shift meant to be maintained for life, even after you all are in your ideal weight range, and are physically active and eating healthfully day in and day out.

Your family doesn't have to be overweight or obese to benefit from this program. Every family member will reap rewards regardless of their weight. Even those who are already doing all they need to do in terms of physical health will benefit from more family togetherness!

How to Calculate Body Mass Index (BMI)

**BMI equals weight in pounds times 703,
divided by height in inches squared.**

BMI is a measurement of weight in pounds divided by height. This measurement can be used to gauge whether it's time to make a stronger effort to lose weight. If your child or another family member has . . .

- A BMI below 18.5, he or she is underweight.

- A BMI between 18.5 and 24.9, he or she is normal weight.

- A BMI between 25 and 29.9, he or she is overweight.

- A BMI of 30 or higher, he or she is obese.

Let's say your child weighs 75 pounds and is 42 inches tall. Multiply 75 times 703, which equals 52,725. Then, figure out 42 times 42 (that's 42 squared), which comes out to 1,764. Divide 52,725 by 1,764, and you get 29.9. If this were your child, he or she would be categorized as overweight, and just on the cusp of falling into the category of obesity. (Some fit, healthy children and adults will fall toward or even the high end of the BMI scale due to genetic predisposition.)

RISKS OF OVERWEIGHT AND OBESITY

About 10 percent of children under the age of six are obese in the United States, and just under 6 percent of infants—babies less than a year old—are obese. Children who start out this way almost always face a lifetime of struggles with their weight. Those who remain at unhealthy weights through childhood and adolescence and into adulthood also face a much greater likelihood of developing chronic diseases, including heart disease, heart failure, arthritis, cancer, diabetes, and asthma, early in their adult lives. The sooner parents can intervene the better.

A child who is overweight or obese is at risk of developing as soon as young adulthood:

- **High blood pressure:** This is directly damaging to blood vessel walls, especially in the heart, and is one of the most important risk factors for heart attacks and strokes.

- **High cholesterol and triglycerides:** High "bad" LDL cholesterol and low "good" HDL cholesterol are linked with increased risk of heart disease; so are high triglycerides.

- **Insulin resistance/type 2 diabetes:** Insulin resistance can lead to high blood sugar, which is damaging to blood vessels and organs throughout the body. Let me explain.

  Carbohydrates from the foods we eat are moved into individual body cells by a hormone called *insulin* after they have been broken down into a simple sugar, glucose, in the digestive tract. This is how individual cells make the energy that powers the body's functions.

  When people are overweight, don't get enough exercise, and have a poor diet, their cells can become *insulin resistant,* meaning that insulin can't any longer move glucose into the cells to make energy. That glucose remains in the bloodstream, leading to high blood sugar (hyperglycemia).

  If insulin resistance isn't caught and reversed with appropriate diet and exercise, the pancreas keeps trying to override insulin resistance by making more and more insulin—and high blood insulin (hyperinsulinemia) is also damaging to blood vessels and organs.

  Eventually, the pancreas peters out and insulin production falls. Then, you've still got high blood sugars but little to no insulin, and this is where a diagnosis of type 2 diabetes is made. Often, there are few or no symptoms of blood sugar imbalances until full-blown type 2 diabetes—with symptoms including unquenchable thirst, extreme fatigue, a browning of the skin called *acanthosis nigricans*, and rapid weight loss—sets in.

Of all the problems that arise from being overweight or obese, diabetes or high blood sugar, high cholesterol, or high blood pressure merit the most concern, especially for heavy children—who are being found to have these problems more and more. About 60 percent of children who are overweight or obese have at least one of these risk factors for heart disease. About 25 percent of this group has two or more of the following risk factors:

- **Bone and joint problems:** Extra weight puts excess stress on knees, hips, ankles, and feet during physical activity. This can predispose a heavy person to developing osteoarthritis at a relatively young age, which can, in turn, make exercising more difficult and pave the way for additional weight gain and health problems.

- **Shortness of breath, asthma, sleep apnea:** Heavy people are more likely to be asthmatic or to have trouble breathing at night. Sleep apnea, where the airway is compressed by excess fat and sleep is interrupted by short periods of not breathing, can make it tough to get a good night's sleep.

- **Earlier sexual maturation in girls, with menstrual/reproductive problems as they grow older:** Fat cells make estrogen, and extra estrogen in the body can lead to early onset of menstruation and breast development. If the idea of a post-pubescent nine- or ten-year-old girl seems a bit scary to you, you're not alone! An overweight or obese girl is also at risk of irregular periods and problems conceiving when she is ready to do so.

- **Social discrimination, teasing, and depression:** One study found that thirteen- to fourteen-year-old obese girls had a fourfold greater risk of having low esteem than girls who were not obese. Low self-esteem leads kids to greater loneliness, sadness, and use of alcohol and tobacco. Overweight and obese children are also at increased risk of depression.

- **Liver and gallbladder disease:** Nine to ten percent of U.S. children have *nonalcoholic fatty liver disease* (NAFLD), where fat collects in liver cells because of a diet too high in unhealthy fats. Eighty percent of these children are overweight or obese. NAFLD can lead to liver failure and the need for a liver transplant. Children with NAFLD are at much greater risk of developing type 2 diabetes.

WHY ARE OUR CHILDREN GAINING SO MUCH WEIGHT?

The causes of all this weight gain are very complex and can be different from person to person. Nonetheless, a few common denominators play a role in just about every case.

A child can be programmed to become overweight or obese even before birth. Some children are genetically more likely to store away extra calories as fat, and to make a lot of fat cells to store them in. Once fat cells are created, they don't go away and fat cells like to be full. This is why a heavy person who loses weight tends to have that weight (and maybe a bit extra) creep back on: his or her body wants to fill up those fat cells.

In the days before processed food, having a body like this was a good thing. It could store away lots of calories (3,500 per pound of fat) when food was abundant, and was more likely to survive in leaner times. But now, in places where plenty of calorie-dense food is always available, these same people who were once genetically gifted are now genetically cursed. They pack on pounds eating the same diet as someone else who is much thinner, and who probably wouldn't have survived a famine 500 years ago.

The environment of the mother's body can also affect a child's risk of obesity. When a baby not born past its due date is born overweight—more than nine pounds at birth—it is often due to the mother being overweight or obese and having either type 2 diabetes or insulin resistance. These moms tend to have chronically high blood sugar, which then puts extra pounds on the baby before it's born. This baby is born wired to pack on more weight, and is at much greater risk of putting on the pounds over successive years.

On the other hand, when a baby is born at low birth weight and then gains weight very quickly over the next months, this can also predispose the baby toward the high end of the BMI charts. This is especially true in babies who are fed formula instead of breast milk.

Many moms see pregnancy as a time to eat as much as they like of whatever they like. They think that gaining a lot of weight during pregnancy is okay. But studies of animal moms have shown that when a rat mother eats a junk-food diet while pregnant, her pups prefer the same kinds of food. It follows that a human mom who eats a lot of sugary breakfast cereal, French fries, ice cream, and cookies may have a child more likely to turn her nose up at fruits and vegetables.

Babies who are breastfed for at least one year, with no supplemental food during the first five to six months, have lower risk of becoming obese or overweight between birth and age five. (A study of about 35,000 female nurses conducted at Harvard Medical School found no connection between breastfeeding as an infant and risk of obesity or overweight past the age of five.)

Once a child starts eating solid food and can feed himself, the real challenges begin. The standard American diet is high in meat, high-fat dairy, and processed foods made from refined grains and sugar, and is sorely lacking in vegetables and fruit. These diets contain very little fiber, "good" fats (more on these later), and vitamins and minerals. They please the taste buds intensely, thanks in large part to the innovations of flavor scientists who create irresistible, almost addictive flavors for processed foods. Although these foods are what nutrition scientists call "energy-dense"— meaning that they pack a lot of calories into not very much food—they do little to satisfy hunger.

We all know that when given a choice, children will gravitate to a bag of chips, a soda, or a burger many times over before they decide it's time to opt for healthier fare. When's the last time your child tossed a head of broccoli in your cart while at the market, just *hoping* you won't tell her to put it back?

Here are a few other factors that often play a role in childhood weight gain.

Advertising

Advertising for less-than-healthy foods has a strong influence, too. According to a study by the Kaiser Family Foundation, children ages eight to twelve see, on average, twenty-one ads for unhealthy foods *every single day*. With so many children surfing the Internet, playing free games, and signing on to social networking sites, they are bombarded with more advertising than ever.

Eating Out Often

Most families spend 40 percent of their family's food budget on food prepared by someone else, outside the home. The average restaurant meal contains far more calories, more fat, and less fiber than the average meal made at home. And these meals tend to taste so good that children will eat more. While cleaned plates might be a rarity at home, children rarely leave much of a McDonald's Happy Meal behind.

Not surprisingly, research from St. Louis University in Missouri has found that families who eat out more, eat fewer fruits and vegetables than families who eat at home more often.

Sweetened Drink Consumption

In the 1940s and 1950s, Americans drank about 10 gallons of soda per person per year. By the 1990s, they were drinking 600 cans per person per year—that's *200 gallons of soda going into one body in a single year*, about half the volume of a standard six-person hot tub.

Although soft drink makers would (and do) argue endlessly about the question of whether this is contributing to the obesity epidemic, the facts are as clear as the cheese puff dust on your child's fingers: it can't be helping to have children consuming 150 or more calories' worth of liquid sugar regularly. Studies actually suggest that liquid sugar is used less efficiently by the body than sugars in solid form. In other words, it's more likely to get turned into fat. And most kids can guzzle a soda *and* eat just as much food as if they'd had some zero-calorie water with their meal. Many studies have found a strong link between sugary drink consumption and risk of children becoming overweight.

Super-sized Portions

Super-sizing options are on a lot of menus, and overall portion size has ballooned. If you decide on the lasagna at Olive Garden, you should know that it packs 1,060 calories and 28 grams of fat. At Ruby Tuesday's, the healthy sounding chicken, pasta, and broccoli dish contains a full day's worth of calories (2,060 calories, 68 grams of fat). A serving of the balsamic vinaigrette dressing at TGI Friday's has 590 calories, before you even pour it over anything. Desserts in these big restaurant chains often contain at least half a day's calories.

While the standard "kids' meal" offered at a restaurant might be smaller in volume and calorie count, it's almost always less nutritious than an adult selection—usually a selection including white-flour pasta, hamburger, hot dog, fries, and maybe a taco or quesadilla in certain parts of the country. A friend told me about one particularly bad restaurant meal her four-year-old son got one night as she and her husband enjoyed salads with salmon—mini-corn dogs in thick, greasy breading, fries, and a soda. And it included dessert—a cup of ice cream. "I could see his little arteries clogging as I sat there," she told me, "and his eyes glazing over from all the sugar!"

In 1957, a fast-food burger weighed, on average, 1 ounce; today, that burger almost always weighs 6 ounces or more. If you ordered a soda with your burger in 1957, it was 8 ounces, but today, that soda is 32 ounces. Then, if you decide to take in a movie after your fast-food dinner, the bag of popcorn you buy will be almost six times bigger than the one your dad bought back in '57 when he went to see *Gunfight at the O.K. Corral*.

Social and Economic Inequality

Healthy food is expensive and getting more so. For some families, it's altogether inaccessible. Inner-city residents often can't get fresh vegetables and fruits at all, and are forced to rely on processed foods, which are far cheaper and can be bought at any convenience store. Families with two working parents often find it impossible to get their children active; they are too busy working one or two jobs apiece just to pay the bills, and children are left to their own devices, sitting in front of screens and eating junk food. In an Associated Press (AP) article on this subject, author Martha Mendoza quotes pediatric endocrinologist Philip Zeitler, M.D., who says that "calorie burning has become the province of the wealthy."

This is a sad truth in the United States: more and more, healthy diets and physical activity are available only to people at higher socioeconomic levels. Children of families who have less income and live in less privileged areas are more likely to be overweight and have related health problems.

The response of government agencies to the obesity problem has been inspiring, but in the case of children's diets, it hasn't been effective. In 2007, the U.S. Department of Health and Human Services and other government agencies spent a billion dollars on nutrition education programs for kids. In a review of fifty-seven of those programs, only four turned out to have any measurable positive impact on the kids who participated. These programs sought to educate children about how to make healthy choices, but for the most part, the kids' taste buds overwhelmed anything they had learned.

One federal pilot program involved giving away fruits and vegetables in school lunchrooms, and the children didn't eat them because they didn't like the taste. Another program offered prizes for eating vegetables and fruits, and that worked for as long as the prizes were available—but as soon as the prizes went away, the kids went back to their chips and sodas.

Parents Setting a Poor Example

The most common mistake parents make in trying to promote healthy diets for their children is not to eat healthy diets themselves. Children follow the example of their parents. If you and your partner aren't walking your talk, know that nothing will change until you do. Endocrinologist Philip Zeitler, quoted earlier, also stated in the same AP article that when children do lose excess weight, it's "because their families get religion about this [weight problem] and figure out what needs to be done."

The "Clean Plate" Policy

Insisting that a child finish everything on his plate overrides his natural ability to know when he's full. Rather than insisting the child should eat whenever it's mealtime or whenever someone puts food in front of him, encourage him to only eat when he's hungry.

Using Food as a Bribe or Reward

Another common error is using sweets or other treats to bribe children into behaving themselves. This creates a lot of confusion for the child, as it links junk food with parental approval and resolution of conflict. Some very health-conscious parents try to exert strong control over their children's food choices, and this seems to backlash causing the child to want those foods more. The opposite goes for offering the child some other reward in exchange for eating a healthy food; it reduces their desire to make healthy choices for the simple reason that they are more healthy.

Sometimes, parents refer to foods as "good" or "bad," and try to totally strike sweets or preferred snacks from the child's diet. This backlashes as well, sometimes driving children to sneak those foods elsewhere and to overindulge when they have access to those treats. Children need to learn to indulge in moderation, just like you do, and to do this, they need some freedom to choose. As someone said, *everything in moderation . . . including moderation.*

Eventually, Mom or Dad, you aren't going to be able to control your child's food choices, so if you are strenuously doing so now, it's time to back off. Strong parental control over food intake has the most impact in three- to five-year-olds, who are then less able to regulate their own caloric intake to match what their bodies truly require.

Lack of Physical Activity

Children age two and older should spend at least one hour per day being physically active. Today, children get less exercise than your dad got as a kid, and less than most of the parents reading this book got in their own childhoods. There are fewer P.E. classes in cash-strapped schools, and those same schools are giving out more homework to children in an effort to help those children excel academically. Neighborhoods and parks are often unsafe for playing outdoors. Children are overscheduled and families' hectic lives don't seem to make room for physical activity.

Too Much "Screen Time"

American children spend, on average, *five hours a day* in front of one kind of screen or another. Children who watch five or more hours of TV a day are over four times more likely to be overweight than those who watch two hours or less a day. Computer, video games, and TV are a constant draw for children, and an alluring solution for parents who have too much to do and little time to engage with their children. Almost half of children ages zero to two are daily TV watchers, despite the American Academy of Pediatrics' recommendation that children under two watch no television at all.

YOU *CAN* HAVE A FIT FAMILY

Now you understand that childhood (and adult!) overweight and obesity has many causes, and that not getting this problem under control could have devastating consequences. You see that reversing this trend requires a multifaceted solution. This is what I'm offering you in these pages.

There are no miracle tricks or get-thin-quick schemes—just the facts, with as much motivation as I can manage without standing there with you, cheering you on.

As a trainer, I know what you need to do in order to get yourself and your children to a healthy weight and into a more energetic, active, healthy lifestyle. As a father, I know that your children watch you like hawks. They're like computers; start programming them at an early age. Raise fitness-loving kids who link being active with fun, loving family time, and they'll never want to stop making those healthy choices. They want you to show them the way through your good example, and nothing else will create any meaningful transformation in your family's health.

In this book, you will find nutritional information with recipes and several family-tested workout programs that are easy and inexpensive. I acknowledge that this kind of transformation is harder for some families than others, but I've done my best to make this advice work for everyone.

The one thing you won't find in here is enough motivation to do what has to be done. No one can talk you into making these changes if you don't truly want them for yourself and your children. You can look over all the scary statistics and still not step up, because stepping up is hard, and it requires time, effort, and a change in thinking—not to mention the commitment to shifting away from some of the dietary and sedentary pleasures you and your family are used to enjoying. This is going to be hard work, but it will also be fun, and it will probably bring your family together in a way you will all enjoy.

Do you want to make excuses, or do you want to do what's necessary to promote the health of your children and yourself? If you've read this far, I think I know your answer.

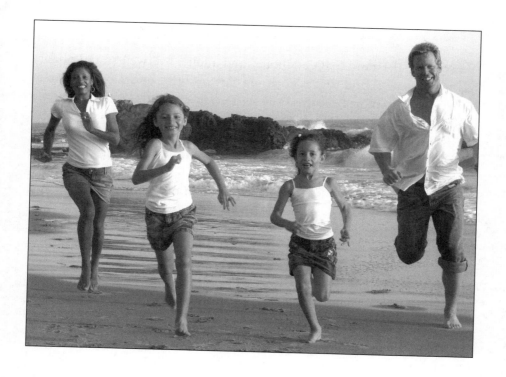

CHAPTER 2

A Really Good Start

Pre-Pregnancy, Prenatal, and Postpartum Nutrition and Fitness

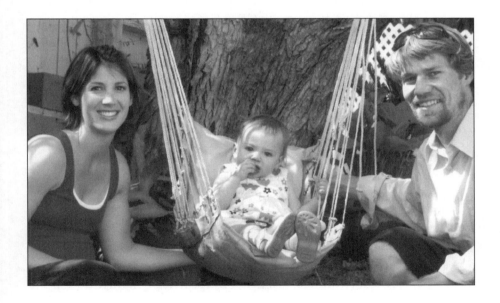

Congratulations! You're pregnant. It's time to put up your feet, eat anything you crave in any quantity you want, and chill for the next nine and a half months . . . right?

I don't think so!

Throughout human history, women have been active all through their pregnancies. We may no longer have to work as hard physically in our everyday lives, but our bodies are still wired to be active—pregnant or not.

You are what you eat, and your baby is what you eat, too. Caving in to every craving for sweets and junk food during pregnancy will, at the very least, probably bring about more weight gain than is ideally healthy and make that hill of losing the baby weight more difficult to climb later on. I'm not trying to stand between you and the occasional Ben & Jerry's celebration or other small indulgences, but overall, your diet during pregnancy—even *pre*-conception, when you are preparing for pregnancy—should be nutrient dense (more on this later) and follow sensible guidelines, which I'll lay out in this chapter.

An easy-to-follow exercise plan will do a great deal for you during and after your pregnancy, whether it's your first or your fifth. Regular workouts promote energy, which is your most needed resource as a mom. It will help improve the health of your heart, control blood pressure, and reduce your chances of developing gestational diabetes, which is most common in women who are overweight or obese. Regular workouts during pregnancy will also help with common pregnancy-related complaints like leg cramps, fatigue, and lower back pain. Getting started on a workout program in the months before conception will help prepare you for a healthy pregnancy and will make continuing to exercise easier. It will become a habit instead of a chore.

Research on women who exercise during pregnancy has found that they tend to have better self-image, better pain tolerance, faster postpartum recovery, and less weight gain (25 percent lower weight gain overall and 50 percent less fat gain) than women who don't exercise during those precious months.

Exercise during pregnancy boosts mood, improves sleep, and reduces aches and pains. And further research shows that in uncomplicated pregnancies, exercise does not increase risk of miscarriage, premature rupture of the amniotic sac, or preterm labor. It lowers the risk of having a baby with very low birth weight.

As long as you follow the guidelines in this chapter, you have no reason to be concerned that exercise will harm your baby. Research shows that prenatal exercise makes for an easier pregnancy and delivery. One study of 500 pregnant women found that the babies of those who exercised had a stronger fetal heart rate and were healthier once born. In this same study, women who exercised regularly spent a third less time in labor. Of those who exercised during pregnancy, 65 percent delivered their babies after four or fewer hours of labor. I've noticed in my pregnant clients—seven so far, including my wife, Nikki—that labor and delivery do seem to go faster for women who maintain their fitness throughout pregnancy.

While this isn't guaranteed—labor and delivery often seem to have their own agendas—having had a prenatal exercise routine will help you maintain your strength and endurance, even if your labor goes much longer than four hours. Giving birth is an endurance event, a strength training session (like no gym workout could ever match!), and a spiritual experience all in one, and it can't hurt to be strong both physically and mentally as you prepare for it.

Pregnancy, too, is a challenge to body, mind, and soul, and taking some time before conception to prepare yourself makes good sense.

PRE-CONCEPTION: SETTING THE FOUNDATION

A pre-conception workout program can be as simple as a daily half-hour walk and some light resistance or weight training two to three times a week. Depending on your level of fitness and whether your doctor feels that weight loss before conception might be in order, you may walk farther or at a higher intensity and do more intense weight training. For guidelines, you can refer to the workouts in this chapter and in Chapter 5, as those workouts are a good place to begin even before pregnancy.

Your diet should consist of as many *whole foods* as possible. A whole food is a food that hasn't been processed. Fill your plate with vegetables, whole grains, and fruit, and use small servings (2 to 3 ounces, or the size of a deck of playing cards) of white-meat chicken, fish, or lean beef. Raw nuts are great sources of good fats and help stave off cravings for sweets.

For more details on the ideal diet for moms at any stage of pre-pregnancy, pregnancy, or postpartum, see Chapter 3. The basics don't change when you get pregnant or after you have the baby, although I will suggest a few adjustments in the chapter on each topic.

Women who classify as obese are more likely to have problems conceiving and to have greater risk of pregnancy complications, neural tube defects such as spina bifida, birth complications, and C-sections (since their babies tend to be larger than average when born). Consult with your gynecologist before conceiving, if possible, to see whether weight loss pre-conception is a good idea for you.

Following the dietary recommendations and workout plans found in Chapters 3, 4, and 5 will help you to lose weight if you haven't been watching your diet or working out. And if you have been, and you're still overweight or obese but fit, rest assured that your body and baby will still reap the benefits of being fit—even if you don't lose all the weight.

If you have any concerns about your baby ending up with peanut or tree nut allergy, avoid eating nuts during pregnancy and breastfeeding, and avoid giving nut butter to your child until he or she is at least three-years-old. (Whole nuts are not recommended for children under the age of five due to choking hazards.)

Prenatal Multivitamins and DHA Supplements

Begin to take a high-potency prenatal vitamin before conceiving if possible. A good prenatal multinutrient supplement will supply your body with iron, which helps prevent anemia (common in pregnancy as mom's blood volume increases); calcium which helps build your baby's skeleton; and folate, a B vitamin folate, which helps prevent certain birth defects.

You may also want to take a supplement made from fish oil, which is rich in a good fat called *DHA* (docosahexaenoic acid). DHA is an omega-3 fat—a "healthy" fat—that is used in the building of a growing fetus' cell membranes, brain, nervous system, and eyes. All the DHA the baby will get for this building project will come from mom's body and diet. Most people living in the United States who eat a standard diet are low on this nutrient, and mothers-to-be are no exception.

Studies of women who have higher intakes or blood levels of this fat during pregnancy than those mothers with low DHA levels have found that their babies:

• Are less likely to be born prematurely.

• Have better attention spans at the age of two.

• Score higher on intelligence tests at the age of four.

Mothers who do what's needed to keep their DHA levels high during pregnancy also seem to be protected against postpartum depression (PPD). In fact, women deficient in DHA and EPA (another omega-3 fat) have six times greater risk of severe PPD and of postpartum obsessive-compulsive disorder. Scientists have done research that suggests that when mom has enough DHA in her body through the years of pregnancy and lactation, her baby may get some protection against eczema, allergies, and asthma.

DHA continues to go to the baby after it's born, through mother's milk. When the mom gets more DHA, more goes into her milk. In different parts of the world, breast milk's content of DHA has been found to vary by more than 100 times. A mother who eats a lot of fish and not much processed food will have much higher DHA content in her milk than one who eats mostly burgers, fries, and high-fat dairy. One study found that of 112 pregnant or nursing mothers, only 2 *percent* were meeting government recommendations for DHA intake.

Children's health expert William Sears, M.D., has said that "DHA is the most important brain-building nutrient at all ages, especially during pregnancy and the preschool years where the child's brain is growing the fastest." Starting with extra DHA during the preconception months will help to build your body's stores in preparation for pregnancy and nursing.

Salmon, sardines, mackerel, and other fatty fish are good sources of DHA. But because of the high level of toxins like mercury and PCBs (polychlorinated biphenyls) in fish, women are being advised to eat fish only two or three times a week, especially if they are considering becoming pregnant or are pregnant already—a sad statement on how polluted our oceans, lakes, and streams have become. (See the inset on page 24 for other species of fish you should avoid or reduce your consumption of.) The issue of overfishing and high food prices also can make it difficult to make fish a regular part of your diet. If you do want to include fish in your diet, choose wild-caught salmon and sardines, which have the lowest levels of toxins.

Dr. Sears suggests that women use a DHA supplement throughout pregnancy and lactation. The amount he recommends is 200 milligrams (mg) per day, but other experts recommend more—up to 2,400 mg per day. The label of the oil should tell you how many milligrams of DHA are in the supplement per pill.

Choose a supplement made from anchovy, sardine, or salmon oils, and

Fish to Avoid

According to the Environmental Working Group, a not-for-profit environmental research organization, *women should avoid eating the following fish when pregnant.* They contain high levels of methylmercury, a chemical that is toxic to the nervous system. Since methylmercury stays in your body for a year and other toxins hang around much longer, it is sensible to avoid them in the months before conception, too.

- Albacore tuna, tuna steaks
- Canned tuna
- Farmed catfish
- Gulf Coast oysters
- Halibut
- King mackerel
- Largemouth bass
- Pike
- Sea bass
- Shark
- Shrimp
- Swordfish
- Tilefish
- Walleye
- White croaker

Eat no more than one serving per month of:

- Blue mussel
- Channel catfish (wild)
- Cod
- Eastern oyster
- Great Lakes salmon
- Gulf Coast blue crab
- Lake whitefish
- Mahi mahi
- Pollock

that has been processed with molecular distillation, which removes heavy metals and other toxins. (Mercury has never been found in fish oil supplements—it doesn't absorb into fat.) Vegetarian supplements made from algae are also available. This algae is the source of DHA added to infant formulas.

Flaxseed and flaxseed oil are often suggested as omega-3 supplements, but they do not contain DHA. They contain another fat that can be transformed into DHA in the body, but the conversion is not very efficient.

Ground flaxseed is great as a fiber source, but to get enough DHA, you will need a supplement made either from fish oil or algae.

HOORAY, YOU'RE PREGNANT!—
AND NAUSEOUS, AND EXHAUSTED, AND . . .

As soon as you cross the bridge between pre-conception and prenatal, you are eating and exercising for two! The advice in Chapters 3 and 4 will keep you on the right track as far as your diet goes. After the first trimester, a pregnant woman requires about 300 calories a day more than a non-pregnant woman. You can expect to gain about a pound a week in a healthy pregnancy.

Dealing with Nausea

If nausea is an issue for you, you may be forced to eat whatever you can tolerate. Most women stop being nauseous by the end of the first sixteen weeks, but some continue to experience this throughout most of their pregnancy. It's called *morning sickness* because it tends to happen in the morning when blood sugar is lowest. But any mom who has been there will tell you that it definitely does not happen only in the morning.

If you have pregnancy-related nausea, you may find it a lot harder to eat a healthy diet, and you'll have to make compromises. If a cheeseburger and fries is all you can keep down, then that is what you will have to eat—don't beat yourself up over it. Keep taking your prenatal vitamins and fish oil. (If you can't keep them down, you might have more success with liquid supplements.)

Most experts believe that morning sickness serves a purpose—probably to protect the baby against naturally occurring toxins in food—and that it is okay to listen to your body's messages about what to eat and what not to eat. Try not to let yourself get too hungry. Nibble crackers, starting first thing in the morning; drink lots of water, thirty to forty-five minutes after meals if it makes you nauseous; sip ginger ale or water with lemon. Try some variations on smoothies made with fresh fruit, yogurt, protein powder, and juice. Some women find that snacks high in protein, such as a slice of cheese or a hard-boiled egg, help prevent nausea from getting out of hand.

If you are nauseous, try to settle your stomach fifteen to twenty minutes before exercising. Have a light snack and see whether you can ease into your exercise session gently (sudden moves can bring nausea back). If all else fails, try to do some light walking and stretching.

Dealing with Fatigue

Fatigue is another common early pregnancy symptom. It usually strikes in the afternoon, and it's a sign from your body that should be listened to—but keep in mind that not exercising can actually make fatigue worse. Schedule time to work out when you tend to have the most energy. Mornings are usually ideal. Or, you can spread your workout into two or three short sessions over the course of the day: a walk in the morning, for example, and light resistance training in the late afternoon.

GENERAL GUIDELINES
FOR THE PREGNANCY WORKOUT

First and foremost, be sure that your obstetrician (OB) or midwife knows about your workout program. Check in with him or her at each appointment to make sure that exercise continues to be safe for you and your baby. (For a list of conditions that could curtail or rule out a prenatal exercise program, see the inset on pages 27–28.)

When doing cardiovascular exercises during pregnancy, keep your heart rate at or below 140 beats per minute. (Around the thirtieth week of pregnancy, your resting pulse will rise about 11 percent, so be prepared to accommodate for this.) The best way to do this is to count your heartbeats for 10 seconds, then multiply by 6. So you're going for a range of about 20 to 23 beats per 10 seconds—that's 120 to 138 beats per minute.

During your cardio workout, check your pulse every few minutes at your wrist, on your neck, or by placing one hand over your heart, and keep moving while you do so, if possible.

Regardless of heart rate, if you find yourself becoming breathless or exhausted, back off. Breathing so hard that you can't carry on a conversation means you're overdoing it. So does a drenching sweat. Light perspiration is fine, but avoid exercising in very hot conditions; if you live in a place

Should You Avoid Prenatal Exercise?

If you have any of the following conditions, the American College of Obstetrics and Gynecology (ACOG) recommends that you be especially careful to consult with your doctor about exercise during pregnancy:

- Addiction to cigarettes (if you still smoke . . . STOP!)

- Anemia

- Asthma (may worsen with pregnancy)

- Diabetes

- Extreme overweight or underweight

- Heart problems or irregular heartbeat

- High blood pressure (a.k.a. hypertension, which may worsen with pregnancy)

- Intrauterine growth restriction (baby grows too slowly)

- Muscle or joint problems (may be made worse by pregnancy-related ligament loosening) or orthopedic problems

- Never had an exercise program before

- Pregnant with multiples (twins, triplets, quadruplets . . .)

- Previous premature labors

- Thyroid problems

- Two or more spontaneous miscarriages

ACOG also has listed some conditions that, if present in a pregnant woman, rule out any exercise program:

- Heart disease

- Incompetent cervix (cervix opens prematurely)

- Lung disease

- Multiple pregnancy at risk of premature labor

- Persistent bleeding during the second or third trimester

- Placenta previa (placenta is not situated properly) after twenty-eight weeks
- Premature labor during current pregnancy
- Preeclampsia or high blood pressure that did not exist before pregnancy
- Ruptured membranes (sac that holds amniotic fluid around the baby has ruptured)

Stop exercising and contact your OB or midwife if, at any time during a workout, you experience:
- Amniotic fluid leakage
- Bleeding
- Calf pain or swelling (may be due to a clot stuck in a leg vein, also called thrombophlebitis)
- Chest pain
- Decreased fetal movement
- Dizziness
- Dyspnea (labored respiration) prior to exertion
- Feeling unusually tired
- Headache
- Extreme muscle weakness
- Premature labor
- Severe abdominal pain

where it gets very hot—up into the high 80s or 90s—try to schedule outdoor exercise early in the morning or late in the evening, when it's cooler, or exercise indoors where there is air conditioning, or in a pool. Dress in layers that you can remove if you become too overheated.

While doing cardio, see whether you can sing "Happy Birthday." If you can sing, you aren't working hard enough!

Ligament Laxity During Pregnancy

Six months into her first pregnancy, a friend of mine went on a steep two-mile hike. She had stuck with an exercise program throughout her pregnancy, and it felt great to hike fast. Then she went home, curled up in her papasan chair and watched a movie on TV . . . and then when it was over, she tried to get up, and her joints hurt so badly that she couldn't get out of the chair without help.

The reason she had this problem is a hormone called *relaxin,* which loosens and stretches ligaments (connective tissue that links bone to bone) to prepare the body to give birth. This especially affects the pelvis, knees, and elbows. It is easy to overstretch or even injure joints with activity that is too vigorous or that involves a lot of fast footwork and direction changes: think tennis, basketball, step aerobics classes. Save the fast footwork and direction changes for postpartum, when your ligaments will tighten again, and take care not to overstretch your joints. See the inset on page 30 for a few body mechanics' pointers for prevention of back injury during pregnancy and postpartum.

Like any workout program, the pregnancy workout includes three kinds of movement: cardio, where you do repetitive whole-body movements to get your heart rate up to or just below 140 beats per minute and keep it there for twenty to sixty minutes; resistance training, where you tone and strengthen muscles throughout the body; and stretching. Cardio and stretching can be done every day, or at least three times a week. The kind of light resistance training you will do during pregnancy can also be done daily; try to fit it in at least two or three times a week.

If fitting twenty- to sixty-minute blocks of exercise into your day seems impossible, go ahead and divide that time into two or three shorter periods spread over the day. You'll get the same benefits you would from doing it all at once.

I've known a few moms who were very fit athletes pre-pregnancy, and had a hard time easing up during pregnancy. One client of mine told me that a friend of hers kept running and doing intense step aerobics classes well into her ninth month. While she didn't have complications from this, this is risky and ultimately not necessary. You can jump right back in only a few weeks after your baby is born. Don't measure your exercise per-

Protect Your Back During Pregnancy and Postpartum

The last thing you need as a pregnant or new mom is to throw your back out. Unfortunately, the demands of pregnancy and caring for an infant can set the stage for this to happen. (Even more so for moms who end up doing both at once, carrying a toddler around while pregnant.) Relaxin makes the low back and the *sacroiliac* joints (joints between either side of the lowest part of the back and the pelvis) much more vulnerable to injury. Here are a few body mechanics' pointers for prevention of back injury during these magical months:

- Lift with your legs! When you have to lift something, bend at the knees and try not to bend at the waist or round the low back. This means squatting down to pick something up off the floor, and it means using your leg muscles to get up from the floor, bed, or a chair.

- When carrying heavy objects, keep them close to your body.

- If you are holding your baby or something heavy in your arms and you have to turn to look at something, turn your whole body instead of twisting at your waist.

- Use a baby carrier instead of holding your baby in your arms all the time. Propping your baby or toddler on one hip—almost always the same hip, for most women—compromises posture and puts your entire spine out of alignment. Soft sling-type carriers, baby backpacks, and many other versions are available (more on this later in the chapter). If you use an over-the-shoulder sling, switch shoulders often to maintain balance. Anytime you hold your baby, avoid tucking your tail down and flattening your lumbar curve; instead, stand tall on your legs and maintain that natural curve in your low back. Don't collapse your chest. Keep your shoulders spread and your breastbone lifted.

- Learn proper nursing technique so that you can bring your baby to your breast instead of hunching forward to bring the breast to the baby.

- Be sure all strollers, changing tables, and other work surfaces are at the right height, so that you can stand up straight. Putting one foot up on a short stool can be helpful when you have to stand for long periods.
- When lifting your baby out of a stroller or crib, bend your knees and keep his body as close to yours as possible while lifting. If you are putting him down on the floor, keep him close to you and don't bend at the waist; instead, step forward with one foot and kneel on the opposite knee to bring him to the floor.
- Postpartum, engage abdominal and pelvic floor muscles any time you have to lift something. This will stabilize your back.

formance during pregnancy against your performance before. If you are already fit when you become pregnant, hold the goal of maintaining your fitness level, not improving it.

PREGNANCY/POSTPARTUM WORKOUT, PART ONE: CARDIOVASCULAR EXERCISE

Walking is the best activity for staying fit or even for improving your fitness during pregnancy and postpartum. All you need is a good pair of running shoes, and it's safe from the first to the last day of a normal pregnancy. In the second half of your pregnancy, I suggest you walk on smooth trails or sidewalks, a track with a cushioned rubber surface, or a treadmill. Loose ligaments and a big unwieldy belly can cause you to lose your balance or injure knees or ankles on uneven surfaces.

When should you return to exercise postpartum? If you have had a C-section, wait until your incision has healed and your OB or midwife gives you the go-ahead to begin exercising. For some women, this will take six to eight weeks; others may need less time. If you had a vaginal delivery, you can get back to exercise as soon as you feel you have enough energy and any vaginal tears or incisions are healed. Check with your health-care provider to make sure you aren't going back to exercise too soon. If you are generally feeling good and continue to feel good after workouts, and if you don't experience discomfort or increased vaginal bleeding, you're ready to start getting back in shape. Some moms need a lot more rest and recovery time, and some need almost none. Only two weeks' postpartum, my wife started walking the track and doing light-freestyle weight workouts three times a week. She was back to her original weight in sixty days!

Moms whose babies are born with health problems could and should hold off; the lack of sleep, extra baby care, and stress of having an ill infant don't need to be compounded with workout obligations. Getting out with your baby for a walk once a day, however, will probably help you maintain your energy and relieve stress. For more good reasons to get out and walk, see the inset below.

Walking

Walking doesn't have to be boring! My wife likes to download workout music into her iPod and jam away during her walks. Other moms I know enjoy listening to podcasts or books on tape while exercising. Go to beaches and lakes, botanical gardens, college campuses, parks, and local trails. Change locations frequently to keep it fresh. See if you can connect with other pregnant or new moms who might like to take walks with you.

Five Reasons a New Mom Should Get Out and Walk Four or Five Times a Week

1. It boosts your energy, which all new moms need.

2. It helps get rid of your "baby weight."

3. It helps reduce or even prevent postpartum depression.

4. It gives you the opportunity to meet and socialize with other new moms.

5. It gets you out of the house, which can be crucial for boosting your confidence during those rough early months.

Swimming and Water Exercises

Swimming and water exercises are widely recommended for pregnant women. You get full-body movement that addresses strength in the core, arms, legs, back, and chest, as well as cardiovascular benefits—with no pounding and very little risk of injury. Pregnant moms also get blissful relief from lugging their big bellies around by passing some time in a cool swimming pool. Since swimming is out of the question for several weeks postpartum, you'll have to take a break from this if it's your preferred mode of cardio.

Keep in mind that swimming has not been shown to be as effective a weight-loss exercise as weight-bearing exercise like walking, dance, or running. Weight-bearing exercise also promotes bone building, which is important during the childbearing years. The more bone you can build during this time, the less likely you will develop osteoporosis later on. If it's something you love, however, or if you have orthopedic problems or are extremely overweight, exercising in the pool may be your best bet.

Prenatal Exercise Class

If you can find a prenatal exercise class where you live, check it out. These classes usually involve some light cardio in the form of low-impact aerobics, gentle strengthening and stretching, and lots of camaraderie with other expectant moms. Usually, there are also educational segments that address labor, delivery, and postpartum questions that mothers often have. This is a great place to find other moms who are invested in exercise and who might want to keep working out together after your babies are born.

Prenatal Yoga

Prenatal yoga is another good option. It builds strength, helps with safe stretching, and teaches breathing and relaxation techniques that can come in handy when the big birth day comes. Prenatal yoga teachers will probably emphasize the need for both strength and relaxation during labor. In the end, I'm told, the birth process requires yielding, relaxing, and letting go just as much as it requires brute strength and endurance, and a good yoga teacher will help you cultivate all these abilities.

Dancing

When my wife was pregnant, she would sometimes put her favorite tunes on the stereo and dance around the living room. She dances all the time, and it seemed a natural progression for her to start dancing with our daughters when they were still growing inside her. It was quite a workout, but never felt that way to her—it was more fun and therapeutic, and gave her a feeling of connection with the baby in her belly. Although I'm not sure about this, I tend to believe that my daughters' inability to sit still any time they hear music has a lot to do with these prenatal boogie sessions. If you decide to try this while pregnant, steer clear of dance moves that involve jumping, twirling, or leaping!

After a workout, you should feel energized, not drained or exhausted. Exhaustion is a sign that you are overdoing it. Getting thirsty, light-headed, or really tired won't be good for you or your baby. For tips on how to stay hydrated, see the inset opposite.

THE "IN-ARMS" PHASE

Postpartum exercising might seem out of the question, because you are now caring for a newborn who seems to have no interest whatsoever in being put into a stroller. Some moms like to time their walks so that their infant falls asleep and naps in the stroller, but you may find that while your baby's napping, you need to be at home taking care of things—or, perhaps, catching some much-needed shut-eye of your own. The way to make this a win-win situation is to use an infant carrier and take your baby with you for walks.

Parents in the United States tend to be over-reliant on strollers. Only since about the middle of the twentieth century have infants been expected to lie still in car seats, cribs, and strollers. Until very recently in human history, babies have been carried and held constantly from birth to at least the point where they can sit up on their own—for most infants, about five to six months of age.

If your baby cries whenever she is put down, keep in mind that she has evolved this way for a reason. She is designed to do the only thing she can do—cry—in order to get herself into someone's arms, where she can be protected and fed. Your instinct to pick that crying baby up is also deeply ingrained. Being held and carried in someone's arms rather than in a car seat or stroller does not "spoil" a baby—in fact, it fulfills important needs in both baby and parent.

A baby who is in-arms or in a carrier that is against mom or dad's body is constantly being stimulated by movement as the adult moves. The baby gets to see the world along with mom or dad and is comforted by the sounds and smells of the parent. A walk can be excellent wide-awake learning and experiencing time for a baby who is carried at a level where she can see what's around her. I will touch more on the importance of holding and carrying your baby in Chapter 6.

Stay Hydrated

When you exercise, your body loses a lot of water. Pregnant moms require extra water (ten 8-ounce cups a day), and breastfeeding moms require even more than that (thirteen 8-ounce cups a day). Even mild dehydration affects muscle power and endurance, and the ability of organs to keep up with the body's demands. Getting adequate water promotes better kidney and liver function (for you and your baby), which is important for cleansing the body of toxins. It can also help alleviate ankle and foot swelling, both common during pregnancy.

Drink two or three 8-ounce cups of water in the two to three hours before you exercise, and drink one more cup just before you begin your workout. Keep a water bottle nearby and sip from it every fifteen minutes or so while you exercise. Then, once you're done, have another two or three cups in the next couple of hours.

Drink at least eight 8-ounce cups of water a day. A reusable, portable water bottle that can hold at least a liter (33 fluid ounces) can help you keep track of your water intake. If your urine is almost clear, you're getting enough.

PREGNANCY AND POSTPARTUM WORKOUT, PART TWO: RESISTANCE TRAINING

Resistance training pits the strength of muscles and tendons against some kind of resistance. That resistance can come from body weight, weight machines, free weights, or elastic tubing. During pregnancy, resistance training is about giving the body enough tone and strength to prevent injury and prepare for labor and giving birth. In the first few weeks postpartum, it's about starting to rebuild strength and reclaim your body. Pregnancy or postpartum—get your doctor's or midwife's okay before doing resistance exercise.

These are the workout moves I recommend for moms-to-be or for those who have recently given birth. The first group of exercises are freestyle moves done without weights; in the second group, a Thera-band (a stretchy rubber band with a handle on each end) is used. Photos of an expectant mom are provided for each exercise to give you a good grasp of proper form. You'll find a beginner and a more advanced version of each exercise.

These resistance workouts are designed to get the full body in motion. Choose one to do twice a week, or mix them up. (Walking and stretching can be done every day.) As you do each exercise, consciously pull up and hold the pelvic floor muscles—the same move suggested in the section on Kegel exercises on page 55.

None of these fifteen- to twenty-minute workouts use weights—you'll just be using your own body weight or some rubber bands with handles. Each repetition should be steady and slow enough to keep every part of the movement controlled by the muscle instead of momentum or gravity.

PREGNANCY FREESTYLE WORKOUT

You'll notice that each of these series of exercises—a freestyle workout that requires no weights or bands at all, a workout that uses a resistance band, and the stretch series—all have nine moves to represent the nine months of pregnancy.

Do ten reps per exercise if you are a beginner and fifteen per exercise if you're more advanced. Beginners can do all nine moves of their chosen workout and call it a workout; more advanced exercisers can do all nine moves, rest for sixty to ninety seconds, and repeat the series one more time.

A week of workouts might look like this:

- Monday: Freestyle workout

- Tuesday: Walk and stretch series

- Wednesday: Repeat Tuesday's workout

- Thursday: Rubber-band workout

- Friday: Repeat Wednesday's and Thursday's workouts (walk, rubber-band workout, and stretch)

- Saturday and Sunday: Family fun!

PREGNANCY/POSTPARTUM FREESTYLE WORKOUT

LYING ABDUCTION

Works the hips and outer thighs.

STARTING POSITION: Lie on your side, head resting on the arm closest to the floor and the other arm bent, hand resting on the floor in front of your chest. Bend the bottom leg slightly and straighten the top leg, keeping the knee and foot pointing straight ahead of you.

ACTION: Press the top leg upward, keeping the hip stacked, as high as it will comfortably go, then lower almost all the way down without relaxing the leg. Repeat 10 to 15 times, then switch legs.

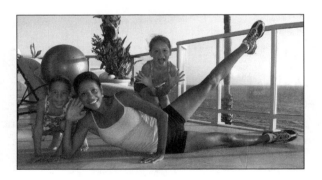

FREESTYLE GOOD MORNINGS

For the hamstrings (backs of legs) and buttocks.

STARTING POSITION: Stand up straight with feet together or six inches apart, hands hanging down. Bend knees slightly and keep them that way throughout the exercise.

ACTION: Keep the back straight and send hips slightly behind you as you lower the hands along your legs to just past your knees, touching your shins with your fingertips. Keep looking out in front of you the whole time and take care not to round the lower back. Then, return to the starting position and shrug your shoulders up toward your ears. Relax the shoulders down before starting the next repetition. Repeat 10 to 15 times.

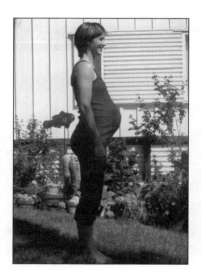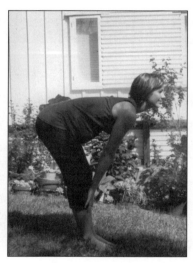

STATIONARY LUNGES + REACH

Works the entire lower body.

STARTING POSITION: Stand tall, feet parallel, arms at your sides. Place your left foot about 3 feet in front of the right. If balance is not an issue, place your arms at a 90-degree angle as you prepare to lunge.

ACTION: Begin bending the front knee and lowering the hips toward the floor while bending the back leg, dipping that knee toward the floor. Make sure your front knee does not move in front of your front ankle and that the front heel stays firmly on the floor. Reach both arms overhead. Then, straighten the back leg and push up, returning to standing position. That's one repetition; bend the back leg again and let the elbows drop again to start the next rep. Repeat 10 to 15 times, then switch to the other leg.

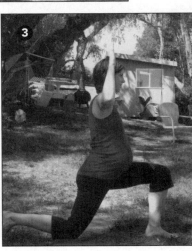
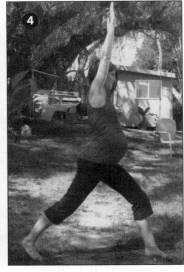
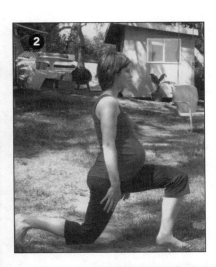
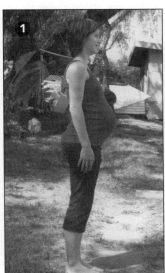

SUMO SQUATS

Works the entire lower body.

STARTING POSITION: Stand with feet more than shoulder-width apart. Many people initially make the mistake of having their feet too close together here, so go ahead and spread them out wide. Let your legs and feet turn out slightly, so that if you brought your feet together they would create a 45-degree angle. You can do this with hands on hips or holding one end of a dumbbell in both hands, so that it hangs straight down in front of your thighs.

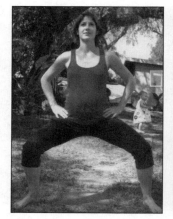 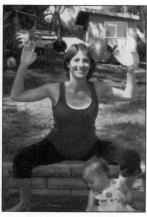

ACTION: Keep looking out in front of you and maintain a natural slight curve in your lower back. Squat down, letting your hips move back as much as they need to in order to prevent your knees from going in front of your toes. Keep your heels on the floor. You can add arms here as shown in the picture: simply raise arms as you bend the knees. To return to starting position, straighten the knees. Repeat 10 to 15 times.

ANGLED PUSH-UPS

Works the chest and triceps (muscles in the back of the upper arms).

STARTING POSITION: You can do this with knees resting on the floor and body in a plank position or standing up with hands on the edge of a sturdy table (as shown in the photo). Either way, place hands shoulder-width apart.

ACTION: Lower the chest down until the elbows are at 90 degrees, then straighten the arms again (without locking the elbows). Repeat 10 to 15 times.

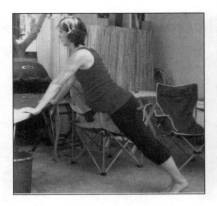
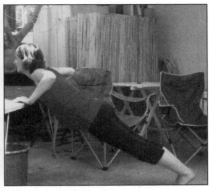

SIDE-TO-SIDE SQUATS

Works the entire lower body.

STARTING POSITION: Stand with feet together or hip-width apart, hands on hips.

ACTION: Step one leg out to the side two to three feet, feet parallel to each other. Keeping hands on hips or reaching arms out in front of you, squat down as though you are trying to sit on a chair placed several feet behind you. Keep looking out in front of you. Return to starting position, then repeat the squat to the other side. Repeat 5 to 10 times per side.

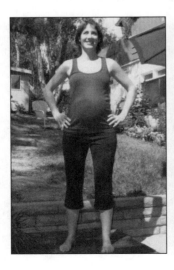
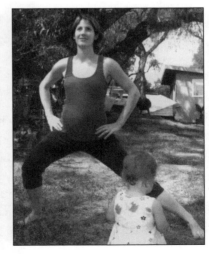

FRONT MATRIX

Works the glutes (muscles of the buttocks) and hamstrings.

STARTING POSITION: Stand with feet hip-width apart.

ACTION: Imagine that you're going to pick up a golf ball that is about three feet in front of you. Step three feet forward with one leg and bend

the knee about 30 degrees. Keeping your spine long and flat, bend forward and reach down to just in front of the front foot with the arm on the same side of your body. Your back heel will come off the floor. If you are pregnant, reach with only your right hand; postpartum, you can reach with both hands. Touch the floor just in front of your foot with the tips of your fingers. Then, push back off the right foot and back into the starting position, all in one smooth motion.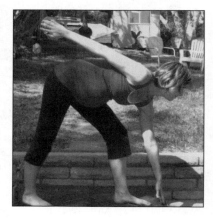

Repeat the move with the left foot stepping forward. Repeat 10 to 15 times on each foot, alternating feet each time.

ROMANIAN GOOD MORNING

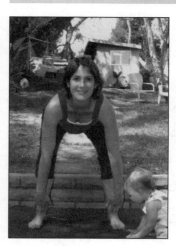

Works the glutes and hamstrings.

STARTING POSITION: Stand with your feet shoulder-width or two to three feet apart. Knees are bent slightly and stay that way throughout the exercise.

ACTION: Keep the back straight and send hips slightly behind you as you lower the hands along your legs to just past your knees, touching your shins with your fingertips. Keep looking out in front of you the whole time and take care not to round the lower back. Then, return to the starting position.

CHAIR SQUATS

More lower body work.

STARTING POSITION: When first trying this exercise, use a chair as a prop. Stand with your back to it, feet hip-width apart. Leave at least a foot of space between your heels and the front chair legs. Once you master the motion, you can do this without a chair, as you never actually sit down in it.

ACTION: Extending your arms out in front of you, sit back until you feel your buttocks just barely touching the chair. Without sitting down, stand back up, dropping your arms back to your sides.

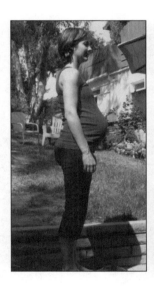 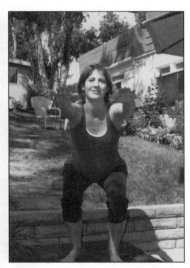

PREGNANCY/POSTPARTUM RUBBER-BAND WORKOUT

This workout uses a Thera-band, a long, stretchy piece of elastic tubing with a nylon handle on each end for easy gripping. You can buy one of these at any sporting goods store. They come in different resistance levels; I suggest that during your pregnancy you use an *easy level of resistance*. Postpartum you can move up to a medium level if you feel the resistance does not offer enough tension.

SQUAT + BAND ROWS

Lower body, upper back, and biceps work here.

STARTING POSITION: Loop the band around something sturdy, like a post, pillar, or the leg of a heavy table. Hold one handle in each hand and back away until your arms are extended out in front of you and the band is taut.

ACTION: This exercise happens in two parts.

First: With feet hip-width apart, squat down, exhaling, until your legs are at a 90-degree angle with both heels planted firmly on the floor; keep looking out in front of you to keep the back flat and long. As you inhale, straighten your knees again.

Second: Then, exhaling again, pull the band's handles toward you, keeping your elbows tucked and shoulders down, until your elbows are behind you and you feel your upper back muscles working. Inhale, let the arms straighten, and on your next exhale, squat again. Repeat 10 to 15 times.

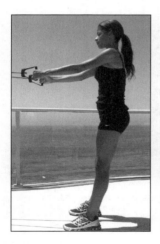 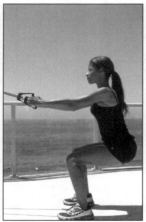 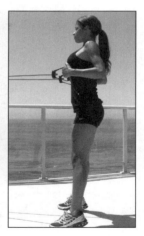

BAND CHEST PRESS

Works the chest and triceps.

STARTING POSITION: Again, loop the band around something sturdy. This time, hold the handles in both hands and turn away from where you have looped the band. Take a step or two away until the band is taut. Hands at mid-chest height, elbows lifted, shoulders relaxed.

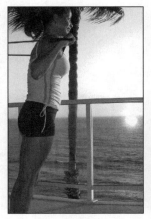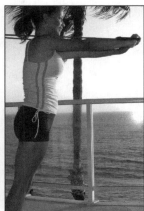

ACTION: Press the handles straight out in front of you until the thumbs meet. Bend the elbows again to return to the starting position. Repeat 10 to 15 times.

SQUAT AND SHOULDER PRESS

Great for the lower body, shoulders, and arms.

STARTING POSITION: Stand with the band looped underneath both feet, holding one handle in each hand. Move your hands up so that they are at shoulder level and elbows are pointing down to the ground.

ACTION: This exercise happens in two parts.

First: Squat the hips down and back, keeping both heels on the floor. Try to reach a 90-degree angle at the knee joint. Then return to the starting position.

Second: Press both hands straight overhead until the elbows are fully straight, then return the hands to the starting position. Repeat 10 to 15 times.

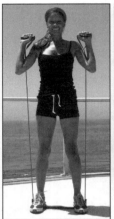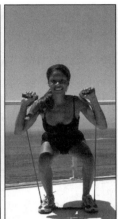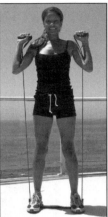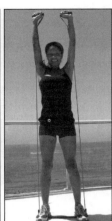

BAND TRICEP EXTENSION

Targets the triceps, on the back of the arms.

STARTING POSITION: Loop the band around something sturdy, like a beam, a pillar, or the top of an open door. Hold one handle of the band in each hand, palms facing down, body in a vertical position, and back away until the band is taut (not tight).

ACTION: Then, with feet together, press both arms straight down along your sides so that your wrists are next to your thighs. Look out in front, keeping your back flat. Then, let your forearms bend, keeping the upper arms totally still, and return to starting position. Repeat 10 to 15 times.

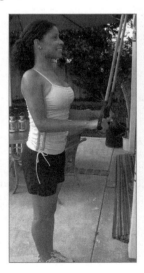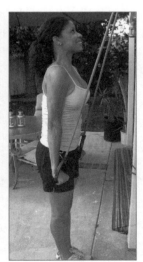

SINGLE-ARM BAND ROW

Works the lats (the long muscles that attach arms to spine).

STARTING POSITION: Wrap the band around something sturdy, like the leg of a heavy table or a pillar. Next stand facing the band or sit on an exercise ball such as a Swiss ball or balance ball, far enough back to make the band taut. Hold the band's handles with palms down.

ACTION: Draw one elbow back along your ribs, pulling it back to just past your torso. Return to starting position and repeat with the other arm. Do a total of 20 to 30 repetitions—10 to 15 reps for each arm.

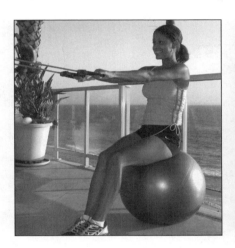 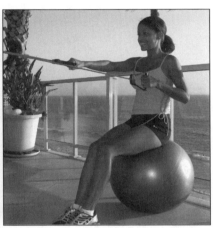

SINGLE-ARM BAND PRESS

The chest and triceps work here.

STARTING POSITION: Wrap the band around a sturdy object behind you. Hold the handles in your hands. Begin with elbows bent, forearms parallel to the ground.

ACTION: This is basically the reverse of the single-arm band rows in the previous exercise, where you do the same motion, but facing in the opposite direction. Press one hand at a time out in front of you, then the other. Do a total of 20 to 30 repetitions—10 to 15 reps for each arm.

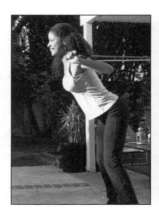
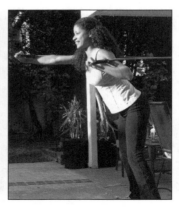

BAND TRI KICKBACK

More targeted work for the triceps.

STARTING POSITION: Attach the band to a sturdy object in front of you. Stand with feet apart, bending at the hips with head up and spine straight. Hold handles with palms down and elbows bent, upper arms along your sides.

ACTION: Press both palms back behind you until your elbows are straight, then return to starting position. Repeat 10 to 15 times.

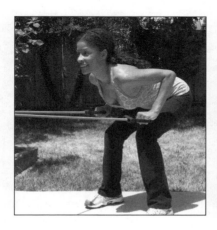
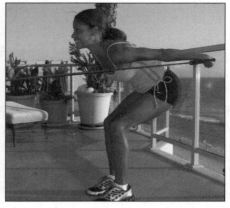

BAND BICEP CURL

Say hello to your tank tops again!

STARTING POSITION: Loop the band under your two feet. Hold one handle of the band in each hand.

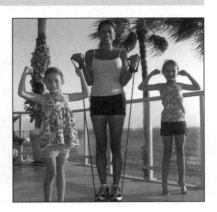

ACTION: Stand tall, lean back a little, and curl your hands toward your shoulders. Keep your upper arms still as you do so. Then, allow the arms to straighten as you return to the starting position. Repeat 10 to 15 times.

SUMO SQUAT + REACH AND CALF EXTENSION

A great combination that works the lower body, core, and calves.

STARTING POSITION: Stand with your feet roughly twice shoulder-width apart. Point your toes outward with your arms bent and hands raised shoulder-height.

ACTION: With head up and torso straight, bend your knees, directing your knees toward your toes, and slowly lowering your hips until your thighs are parallel to the floor. Return to standing, reaching your arms straight up, until your legs are straight; then rise a little higher by coming up onto the balls of your feet. Try to hold for 1 to 2 seconds, then return to flat feet to begin the next repetition. Repeat 10 to 15 times.

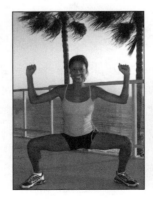

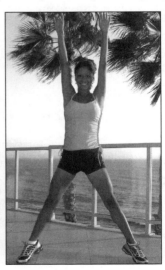

PREGNANCY/POSTPARTUM STRETCH SERIES

Regular stretching has many benefits. It helps to reduce muscle tension, improve circulation, reduce stress, and decrease risk of injury. During pregnancy, these benefits include preparation of the pelvic and thigh muscles and pelvic ligaments for labor and birth. Back pain, which is very common in pregnant women and in new mothers who lug fast-growing babies everywhere they go, can be prevented with a good stretching program.

Because of the effects of relaxin, pregnant moms may find that they can stretch more deeply than they could before. If this happens to you, be cautious, because you can overstretch and injure muscles, tendons, or ligaments. A few pointers for stretching during pregnancy:

- Avoid quick, jerky, or bouncy movements during stretches; go slow and easy.

- Move into a stretch to your "edge"—the point where you feel it pulling strongly, but not to where it hurts. Often, people think that if they can't touch their toes in a hamstring stretch, they aren't doing it right. Everyone has different levels of flexibility; the point is to align your body so that you are feeling the stretch in the right part of the body, go to that edge and stay there for a few breaths.

- Stretch after exercising, when your body is warmed up completely.

Last but not least are nine pregnancy-stretching moves. Hold each stretch for 30 to 60 seconds, breathing deeply and relaxing your body.

LOWER BACK STRETCH (CHILD'S POSE)

STARTING POSITION: Come onto all fours on a mat, carpet, or other soft surface with the tops of your feet against the floor. Spread your knees wide enough to make room for your belly.

ACTION: Sit back onto your heels and fold forward over your legs, putting your forehead on the floor. (If this feels uncomfortable, you can cross your arms on a pillow and rest your forehead on your arms.)

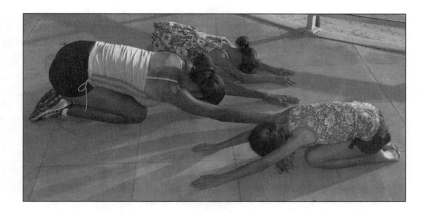

HIP FLEXOR STRETCH

STARTING POSITION/ACTION: Come to the floor on all fours. Step one leg forward between your hands, bringing that leg to about a 90-degree angle as you gently lunge your other leg behind you. Keep both hands on the ground on either side of your front foot. Either place the 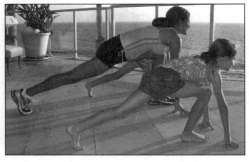 knee of the back leg on the floor, or press that knee straight for a deeper stretch. Tuck your tailbone down and let your hips sink with each exhalation. Hold for 30 to 60 seconds, then repeat on the other side.

BUTTERFLY STRETCH

STARTING POSITION/ACTION: Stand with feet spread wide and toes slightly turned out. Then, squat deeply, keeping both heels on the floor. (You may have to adjust your feet to get a deep enough stretch.) If your calves are tight and your heels pop up, you can place a long, rolled-up towel or blanket beneath your heels for support. Clasp your hands between your legs, then place your elbows in your inner knees and use your elbows to press your knees open as you sink into the stretch. (See next page.)

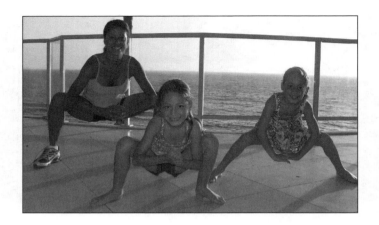

ANGRY CAT STRETCH

STARTING POSITION: Begin on your hands and knees on a soft surface, with knees directly below hips and hands directly under shoulders. Your spine begins in a neutral position.

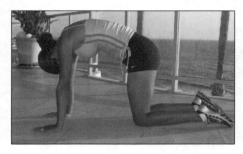

ACTION: Inhale, tucking your chin into your chest and drawing your lower abdomen in toward your spine as you round your back. Exhale as you return to the starting position.

INNER THIGH STRETCH

STARTING POSITION: Stand with feet slightly wider than hips. Turn your toes outward slightly.

ACTION: Lunge to one side, bending the knee on that side and straightening the other knee. If you can reach the floor with your hands, do so, coming to about a 90-degree angle in the bent knee and sending your tail out behind you. If you're not comfortable reaching for the floor, place your hands on your hips or on the back of a chair, but still think about sending your tail behind you—this will help you to get the deepest stretch in the inner thigh.

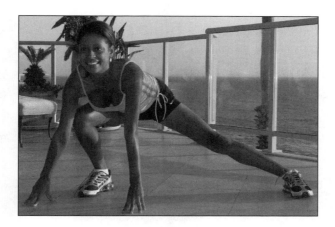

SEATED LEGS-APART HAMSTRING STRETCH

STARTING POSITION: Sit on the floor with legs extended out in front of you. Slide your legs as far apart as you comfortably can while still keeping your torso upright and shoulders relaxed. (If this feels very difficult, sit on a pillow or a folded blanket to elevate your hips above your feet.)

ACTION: Place your palms on the floor in front of you. Slide your hands out in front of you and bend forward. Keep your knees and toes pointing straight up toward the ceiling.

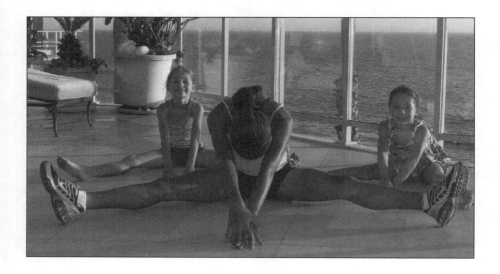

STANDING QUAD STRETCH

STARTING POSITION: If you want help with balance, do this one next to the back of a chair or a wall.

ACTION: Reach behind you with one hand to grab the foot or ankle on the same side of your body. Press the thighs together, aiming the knee of the lifted leg toward the floor. Tuck your tail to lengthen the front of the hips as you hold the stretch. Repeat on the other side.

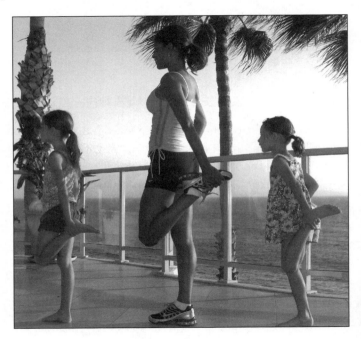

STANDING HAMSTRING STRETCH

STARTING POSITION: Stand facing the seat of a low table, chair, stool, or step. Carefully place the heel of one foot onto the table/chair/stool/step (using another wall or chair for balance if necessary). Slightly bend the standing leg and press your tailbone up toward the ceiling.

ACTION: Keeping your torso straight, fold your upper body toward the extended leg, bending from the hips. Hold for 30 seconds.

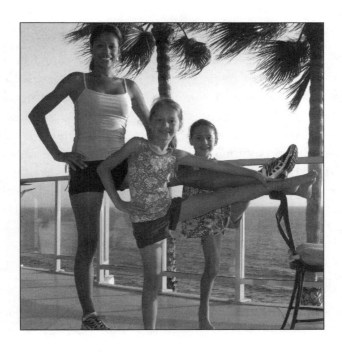

After the first trimester, avoid any exercise that requires you to lie flat on your back. The extra weight of the baby on blood vessels in the belly reduces blood flow both to the baby and to the mother's heart and brain.

Squeeze More Kegels into Your Day

This exercise helps to tone and strengthen the vaginal walls and pelvic floor. Strengthening these muscles is great preparation for giving birth and an important part of preventing that common postpartum issue of sneeze-induced, cough-induced, or laughter-induced leakage of urine. Start doing them during pregnancy, if possible, or at least postpartum, and continue for the rest of your life.

Here's how to do them: contract the muscles you would contract if you were trying to stop urinating. You should feel this in your vaginal walls. Pull upward and inward. Hold for a count of three, then slowly relax. Aim to do fifteen each day, working toward lengthening each hold to a count of five, and then to a count of ten. Driving in your car, watching TV, standing in line at the market or bank—you can do these anywhere!

CONCLUSION

If you are more inclined to sit on the couch with your feet up than to exercise while pregnant or postpartum, remember: the big demands of motherhood will be easier if you are physically strong. Carrying a baby around nearly all day for months will take a toll on your back, neck, and shoulders, if you don't stay strong in your core and limber in your joints.

The most important things you can do during the first weeks' postpartum: care for your baby, rest when possible, and eat a healthy diet. Time for exercise will come soon enough, so don't feel you need to push too hard too soon. Listen to your body and do workouts that feel good.

CHAPTER 3

Fit Family Food Fundamentals

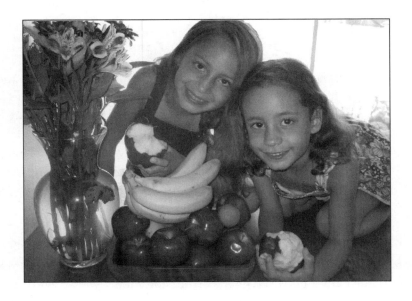

While children's nutritional needs are somewhat different from those of their parents, the fundamentals are the same for people of all ages. Following these guidelines may require major changes in the way your family eats and in the way you shop for food.

Don't worry—in Chapter 4, you will find a sample Fit Family Food Plan, complete with shopping list, that you can create variations on as you go. In the back of the book, you'll find some recipes to help you shift to a healthier way of feeding your family—and yourself. Chapter 4 will also give specific guidelines for feeding children from infancy into their elementary school years in ways that will set the stage for a lifetime of healthful eating.

In this chapter, I'll share some more general tips for a Fit Family Diet.

THE FUNDAMENTALS

If you adhere to these general guidelines, you'll find yourself eating a more nutritious diet. Not only will this help your baby get proper nourishment while in utero, but also it will help your body make plenty of nutrient-dense milk and will aid you in shedding baby weight when the time comes. These tips will see you through your children's early years as well, helping you to set dietary rules in your home that will give them the best possible start.

Go Organic When Possible

Children and pregnant women are advised to eat organically grown foods whenever possible. The small bodies of children concentrate pesticides and other chemicals more quickly than those of adults, so they can tolerate less of these chemicals before they affect their bodies and brains. Pesticides are known to cross the placenta and pass into the growing body of the fetus, and early evidence shows that this may affect fetal growth. Researchers at the University of Washington, Seattle, found six times the level of specific pesticides in the urine of preschoolers who ate conventionally raised foods than in the urine of classmates who ate mostly organic.

Women who are breastfeeding should also try to choose organic foods whenever they can. Toxins from the nursing mom's diet pass into her milk and into her baby's body. Pregnant or nursing moms who wish to try to reduce the toxicity of their breast milk may find some answers in a book by Robert Rountree, M.D., and Melissa Lynn Block entitled *The New Breastfeeding Diet Plan: Breakthrough Ways to Reduce Toxins & Give Your Baby the Best Start in Life* (McGraw-Hill, 2006).

Energy In Should Equal Energy Out

Calories consumed should not exceed calories expended, but with nursing infants and toddlers, calorie counting is totally unnecessary—it's all about feeding the child the right kinds of food. If you do this and encourage physical activity, caloric intake will take care of itself. The child's body is capable of regulating caloric intake—even if he eats more on some days, he'll naturally eat less to compensate on other days.

Having said this: when it comes to sweets, breads, and cereals, serving sizes can be deceiving, and natural appetite can be trumped by powerful, sweet tastes.

In other words, it's far easier and more pleasurable to eat 500 calories' worth of bread or cookies than to eat the same number of calories' worth of vegetables or fruits. A single bagel with cream cheese or a pastry can easily amount to 500 calories, but you'd have to eat eight apples, or eight cups of melon, or twenty-five cups of zucchini to reach the same calorie count!

Refined flour foods are calorie dense and tend to be low in nutrient density, unless they are serious nuts-and-berries whole-grain varieties. The average store-bought bagel, for example, equals three or four of the U.S. Department of Agriculture's (USDA) standard servings for grains and can pack 300 to 400 calories—before you even put the cream cheese on top! Even a toddler can easily plow through one of these fluffy white-flour bagels at a sitting. The same goes for muffins, which were once about 1 to 2 ounces and now average about 8 ounces—enough grains for a young child for the entire day.

Also: read labels on packaged foods. Many chips, cookies, sugary drinks, and other treats contain more than one serving per container, and a child will usually be glad to consume the whole thing.

Easy Serving Size Estimation

Unless you have a food scale handy, the recommendation to eat an ounce of something may not be a practical one; still, most guidelines for daily servings use this unit of measurement. Since serving size often is difficult to control, it's important for parents to have at least a ballpark idea of what to look for. Here, on the following page, from registered dietician Frances Largeman, are some easy ways to measure serving sizes of foods commonly eaten. You might consider photocopying this chart and posting it on your refrigerator for easy reference.

NUMBER OF SERVINGS/AMOUNT RECOMMENDED FOR EACH FOOD GROUP PER DAY, BY AGE

VEGETABLES

AGES 2–3: 1 cup   **AGES 4–8:** 1.5 cups   **AGES 9–13:** 2 cups   **TEEN–ADULT:** 2.5 cups

FRUITS

AGES 2–3: 1 cup   **AGES 4–8:** 1–1.5 cups   **AGES 9–13:** 1.5 cups   **TEEN–ADULT:** 2 cups

GRAINS

AGES 2–3: 3 oz. (1 oz. equals a slice of bread, $1/2$ cup cooked cereal, $1/2$ cup rice or pasta, or 1 cup cold cereal)

AGES 4–8: 4–5 oz. (1 oz. equals a slice of bread, $1/2$ cup cooked cereal, $1/2$ cup rice or pasta, or 1 cup cold cereal)

AGES 9–13: 5–6 oz. (1 oz. equals a slice of bread, $1/2$ cup cooked cereal, $1/2$ cup rice or pasta, or 1 cup cold cereal)

TEEN–ADULT: 6 oz. (1 oz. equals a slice of bread, $1/2$ cooked cereal, $1/2$ cup rice or pasta, or 1 cup cold cereal)

MEATS/FISH/BEANS/NUTS

AGES 2–3: A total of 2 oz. from any combination of the following: 1 oz. meat, poultry, or fish; 1 tbsp. nut butter; 1 egg; $1/4$ oz. cooked beans; or a small handful of nuts or seeds (only in children who chew well and won't choke)

AGES 4–8: 3–4 oz. from any combination of the following: 1 oz. meat, poultry, or fish; 1 tbsp. nut butter; 1 egg; $1/4$ oz. cooked beans; or a small handful of nuts or seeds

AGES 9–13: 5 oz. from any combination of the following: 1 oz. meat, poultry, or fish; 1 tbsp. nut butter; 1 egg; $1/4$ oz. cooked beans; or a small handful of nuts or seeds

TEEN–ADULT: 5.5 oz. from any combination of the following: 1 oz. meat, poultry, or fish; 1 tbsp. nut butter; 1 egg; $1/4$ oz. cooked beans; or a small handful of nuts or seeds

DAIRY PRODUCTS OR OTHER CALCIUM-RICH FOODS

AGES 2–3: 2 cups of dairy (milk or yogurt) or dairy alternative (such as calcium-fortified orange juice or soy milk/soy yogurt) or 2 oz. cheese, or mix and match (e.g., 1 oz. cheese, 1 cup milk)

AGES 4–8: 2 cups of dairy (milk or yogurt) or dairy alternative (such as calcium-fortified orange juice or soy milk/soy yogurt) or 2 oz. cheese, or mix and match (e.g., 1 oz. cheese, 1 cup milk)

AGES 9–13: 3 cups of dairy (milk or yogurt) or dairy alternative (such as calcium-fortified orange juice or soy milk/soy yogurt) or 3 oz. cheese, or mix and match (e.g., 1.5 oz. cheese, $11/2$ cups milk)

TEEN–ADULT: 3 cups of dairy (milk or yogurt) or dairy alternative (such as calcium-fortified orange juice or soy milk/soy yogurt) or 3 oz. cheese, or mix and match (e.g., 1.5 oz. cheese, $11/2$ cups milk)

Source: Largeman, Frances, "Portion Control," DiscoveryHealth.com, http://health.discovery.com/centers/nutritionfitness/nutrition/articles/expert/largeman/portioncontrol.html, accessed July 23, 2008

SERVING SIZE REFERENCE	
1 oz. of grains	1 slice of bread, $1/2$ cup cooked cereal, $1/2$ cup of rice or pasta, or 1 cup cold cereal
1 serving of cheese	1.5 oz., or the size of three dominoes
3 oz. of meat	Size of a deck of playing cards or of the palm of an adult's hand
Vegetarian protein sources	$1/2$ cup of cooked beans or 2 tbsp. of nut butter (a serving about the size of a golf ball) are equivalent to 1 oz. of meat
1 serving of leafy greens	Size of a baseball
1 serving of cooked vegetables	Size of half a baseball or a 6-oz. glass of vegetable juice
1 serving of chopped fruit	Size of half a baseball
1 serving of whole fruit	Size of a tennis ball

Source: Largeman, Frances, "Portion Control," DiscoveryHealth.com, http://health.discovery.com/centers/ nutritionfitness/nutrition/articles/expert/largeman/portioncontrol.html, accessed July 23, 2008

Keep in mind that almost every child will go through periods of hardly eating at all, alternating with periods of eating huge amounts of food. Don't force the issue if your baby or toddler isn't interested. She will be soon enough.

Keep Junk Out of the House

You, the parent, control what foods come into your home. You can also be the one to control when those foods are available. Children will get used to eating from whatever's around, although they may complain when their favorite treats aren't around anymore. (It's okay to buy those treats once in a while to help your kids feel less deprived.)

Whole Foods Are "Anytime Foods"

Foods most eaten should be nutrient-dense whole foods. This includes vegetables, fruits, whole grains like brown rice or oatmeal, nuts, eggs, lean poultry, seafood, or tofu. A nutrient-dense diet contains a lot of vitamins, minerals, fiber, and healthy fats per calorie. With your child, you can call these foods "anytime foods."

Whole foods are almost always low in caloric density. Research has shown that diets that contain more low-caloric-density foods (especially foods rich in water like soups, vegetables, and fruits) spur faster weight loss than those that don't make a point of recommending these kinds of foods.

Don't Cut Out the Fat . . .

"Low fat" does *not* equal healthy. In fact, the most recent evidence shows that monounsaturated fats from olive, canola, and peanut oils, and polyunsaturated fats from soy, corn, and sunflower oils are good for our health. Fats from fish are also healthful, and both adults and children can use fish oil supplements if they don't like seafood.

Small children need fat and cholesterol in their diets. Don't feed them low-fat foods (aside from low-fat dairy foods after age one; if you are using organics and your child is within normal weight ranges, you can give them full-fat dairy) and don't restrict their intake of healthy, whole-food-based cholesterol or calories. Choose healthful sources of fats: poultry, eggs, vegetable oils (especially olive), fish, plain yogurt, and nuts over fatty cuts of red meat or cured or highly processed meats, such as bacon, sausage, ham, jerky, and lunch meat.

. . . Or the Carbs

Children should never be placed on a low-carb or no-carb diet. They require plenty of carb-based energy . . . but that energy should come from whole-grain products, vegetables, and fruits as often as possible.

Don't Put Your Kid on a "Diet!"

Adults seem constantly swept into dietary fads that involve extreme changes. While these diets can work for weight loss in the short-term for these grownups, I strongly suggest that you not try to impose these kinds of restrictive, unbalanced diets on a child of any age, and that you set a good example by avoiding them yourself.

It's best not to talk to a child about "going on a diet" or having to lose weight, but simply to shift to improved patterns of eating and activity because this is what is best for the whole family's health.

No diet plan that brings about rapid weight loss is likely to bring about *lasting* weight loss. Only a long-term commitment to a healthy eating plan will have this effect. Don't send your children a message that getting thin quick is the answer. It's harmful to the child's self-image, and doesn't work in the end.

A very interesting study came out while I was writing this book: it involved 314 pairs of parents and overweight teens who signed up to answer some survey questions with researchers at the University of Minnesota. The parents were asked whether or not they knew their child was overweight. Then, they were asked whether they had changed the family diet, had started to eat more family meals and watch less TV during those meals, and had encouraged their child to be more physically active or to go on a diet.

The only difference in the answers between parents who *knew* their teen was overweight and those who claimed they *didn't* know: the parents who knew their teen had a weight problem were more often encouraging their kids to diet. I wasn't surprised to find that those kids, five years later, weighed *more* than they had when the questionnaires were first filled out.

Help Your Child Establish a Healthy Relationship with Food

You want your child to see food first and foremost *not* as an enemy, but as fuel for growth, strength, smarts, and energy. Children need to be taught to see their appetites as healthy, not as something to be suppressed, ignored, mastered, or controlled. Children's relationship with food is best when it adheres to their bodies' natural needs and when it comes back to gratitude for the gifts of nature and the great tastes of wholesome food.

It's best when families cook and eat together at least nightly and participate together in meal planning and shopping, because this embraces food as a central and positive aspect of family life. The family meal is so important that I've devoted a good deal more space to it in Chapter 6, "Fit Family, Smart Family, Happy Family."

Allow Your Child to Choose What to Eat from the Foods You Offer—Or to Not Eat at All

Do your best to offer *something* that the child is sure to like: maybe some whole-grain bread or crackers with nut butter, veggies with dip, or cubes of cheese with apple slices. Your child may well choose to not eat at all if he doesn't like what you're offering, and one day, you may find that suddenly his old favorites are no longer acceptable. That's okay—he won't starve.

Encourage Your Child to Try New Foods— And to Try Old Foods Again

A child will go through phases of liking certain foods and then rejecting them. Remind your child that taste buds change, and that a food he didn't like before may be delicious to him now. It may take several tries before a child will accept a new food into his diet.

Highly Processed Foods Are "Sometime Foods"

Sweets, refined calorie-dense grain products (white bread, white pasta, crackers, pretzels, etc.), sweetened drinks, red meat, chips, high-fat dairy products, and butter should be consumed with extreme moderation. Tell your child these are "sometime foods" that they can have once in a while— maybe two or three times a week.

Some families get around the nag factor (and teach days of the week) by making these choices available only on certain days: for example, only on Fridays and Saturdays, or only on weekends.

Don't Give Juice Right Before Dinner

Juice is calorically dense and can give your child a feeling of being full before sitting down for the family meal. Offer only water before dinner.

Avoid Trans Fats Completely

Hydrogenated vegetable oils, which contain trans fats, should be avoided completely. Trans fats are terrible for your arteries and are implicated in heart disease more strongly than even that old culprit, saturated fats. Food labels now have to state whether they use this kind of oil, but the government does not require them to state any amount of trans fat under half a gram. A food that includes "partially hydrogenated oil" or "hydrogenated oil" in its list of ingredients but that says it has zero grams of trans fat probably skates just below that half-a-gram limit. Avoid it.

TIPS AND TRICKS FOR FAMILIES

Here are a few small pointers that can make a big difference in the way families eat, once the kids are at least three-years-old:

- Put out a platter of fresh, cut-up vegetables with a healthy dip (such as an organic salad dressing or yogurt dip) just before lunch or dinner, when the kids are hungry.

- Keep a bowl of fresh, washed fruit available, within reach of little hands.

- Take snacks or lunch along when you go on an outing instead of stopping for fast food. Pack healthful treats like cashews, dried fruit, celery sticks filled with almond butter and raisins, nut butter and banana sandwiches on whole-grain pita bread drizzled with honey, or whole-grain quesadillas made with apple slices and a small amount of grated sharp cheddar cheese.

- Always take water along on outings so that you don't end up buying sugary drinks for your children when they're thirsty.

- Begin to put out a little extra effort to make children's foods visually appealing once they are old enough to feed themselves. Let your creativity go wild! Cut vegetables and fruit into fun shapes; make "nibble trays" with compartments containing different finger foods and soft foods; cut a soft sandwich of whole-grain bread, nut butter, and no-sugar-added preserves into fun shapes; give the child a toothpick to eat cubes of cheese or cut-up bits of grape.

- Some children enjoy cutting up their own food. Offer a knife (not too sharp, of course!) to a toddler or preschooler who wants to cut up soft foods like banana or cheese. Some kids may also enjoy making their own nibble trays.

- Don't try to force, bribe, or threaten a child into eating any food. It rarely works, and even when it does, it sets up an adversarial relationship between the child and the food that tends to escalate. Let it go, and keep bringing it back.

- Think of ways you can incorporate less-likeable vegetables so your child will enjoy their flavors. Try blending them with others they like more. Chopping, grating, or pureeing vegetables can help you "hide" them if you have a child who tends to pick out or eat around anything that looks green. For example: you might add pureed butternut squash or cauliflower to macaroni and cheese, or finely chopped spinach or grated zucchini (squeeze out extra liquid before adding) to tomato meat sauce made with ground turkey.

- Make smoothies for your kids using plain yogurt, frozen fruit, and small amounts of juice or milk. These can be frozen in paper cups with a Popsicle stick inserted when the mixture is slushy to make healthy Popsicles.

- Consider growing your own vegetables and fruits. Children who almost always eat homegrown veggies and fruit are more than twice as likely to eat their "five a day" than children who eat no homegrown produce. Children who start eating homegrown produce from an early age have a much stronger preference for vegetables and fruit than do other children. If you don't want to garden at home, talk to other parents at your child's school or in your neighborhood about a community garden. Check out the website of the American Community Gardening Association: www.communitygarden.org.

Talk to Your Child about Fast-Food and Junk-Food Ads

Let's say your child comes running to you from the TV room, shouting about some new fast-food meal or kid-friendly snack he has seen a commercial for. "I want it! I *have* to get it!" he hollers. This is a prime opportunity for you to talk to him about junk-food and fast-food advertising.

Make it clear to the child that there is a difference between a TV program and a commercial; that the commercial is about persuading them to buy a product (or, as it usually happens, to persuade the child to try to persuade his parents to buy it for him). The non-partisan organization Common Sense Media (www.commonsensemedia.org), dedicated to improving the media lives of kids and families, suggests that parents ask the following questions when this comes up (adjusted, of course, to the age of the child):

1. Why do you think the advertiser put this commercial on this program? *This will help you to show the child that the advertiser knows that kids like him are watching, and they want to sell their product directly to him through that influence.*

2. Why do you think the commercial uses catchy music or slogans? *This helps the child see how advertisers manipulate children to push their products.*

3. What's appealing to you about this commercial? *Brings #2 deeper by letting the child figure out how the commercial has gotten him to want that particular product.*

4. What might the advertisers be leaving out of the commercial? *If you have been talking to your child about "sometime" and "anytime" foods, encourage her to talk about why this is a "sometime" food. Does the advertiser tell about why the food is healthy for her body? Is it really?*

5. Does it make a difference to you that a celebrity or cartoon character was on the commercial? *This encourages the child to see how the advertiser uses the celebrity testimonial—or simply the "opinion" of the actor who appears in the commercial—to try to sell something.*

ENJOY YOUR FOOD, ENJOY YOUR FAMILY

In the end, don't think that eating healthy means a Spartan diet and no treats. You and your children can enjoy reasonable servings of treats and favorite foods—even junk foods—in moderation, in the context of an overall healthy diet. If your child has that sweetened fruity yogurt or other junk food and suddenly wants nothing else, don't fear; just get back on track with the foods you know are best for you and your family.

CHAPTER 4

Fit Family Food Plan

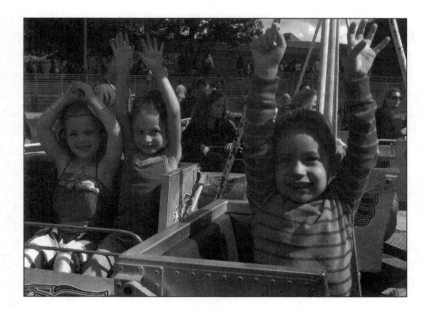

Ever hear about that study on children and eating, where hungry kids were set loose in a room where sweets and junk food were set out along with healthy foods to see what they would choose? Initially, the story goes, the children gravitated to the sweets and junk, and ignored the healthy choices. But after a few bouts of gorging on the bad stuff, supposedly these children started to naturally choose what was good for them—what their growing bodies truly needed.

As far as I can tell, this is an urban myth. Any parent of a child old enough to say "no" to a plate of broccoli knows that most young children won't make healthy choices on their own, as long as delicious but unhealthy choices are available. That they go through phases where they flatly refuse to eat anything that isn't made from white flour, or where they want one food and one food only, or where nothing but dessert holds their interest.

After repeated arguments, battles, tantrums, pleas of "Just try a taste," threats, and bribery, many parents throw up their hands and start feeding their kids nothing but "kid-friendly" foods: mac and cheese, white-flour pasta with butter, peanut butter and jelly on white bread, chicken nuggets, sweetened breakfast cereal or sweet yogurt, hamburgers, hot dogs, fries. Some even resign themselves to preparing separate meals for their children at dinnertime.

In this chapter, we will look at ways you can avoid this outcome by setting healthy eating patterns for your infants, toddlers, and preschoolers.

Keep in mind that no attempt to get your child to eat healthy is going to succeed if they don't see *you* enjoying those foods you want them to eat. But before we get into the topic of solid food, let's look at what is probably the most important food your child will ever consume: breast milk.

BREASTFEEDING FOR A BABY'S BEST START

Back in the late 1960s and early 1970s, only 25 percent of American women breastfed at all. Today, more than 68 percent of new mothers breastfeed their newborns. This is a huge improvement, and is likely to bring improvements in the health of this up-and-coming generation.

Breastfeeding's benefits to baby and mother are well known. If you are a mom-to-be or a new mom, you have probably learned about them already, but let's do a quick listing for those who might not know them all.

I know that some women start out totally convinced of these benefits, and then end up switching to formula because of nursing problems. Far be it from me to judge those women—some women can't nurse their babies for one reason or another. Thank goodness that we have such good, safe formulas for the babies whose mothers have trouble with nursing.

Formulas are better than they have ever been, so mothers who need them can have faith that their babies are adequately nourished. I list breastfeeding's benefits below not to guilt-trip moms who have already made the choice to switch to formula, but to convince those who are on the fence about nursing because they don't fully grasp the benefits to mother and baby.

Breastfeeding Benefits

For Baby

- Reduced risk of infections, including ear infections, tonsillitis, urinary tract infection, flu, pneumonia, and gastroenteritis (digestive infection that causes diarrhea), because of immune factors in breast milk.

- Higher IQ (at ages eight, twelve, and eighteen, children who were breastfed scored 10 to 12 points higher on IQ tests than those who got formula).

- Better visual acuity.

- Greater acceptance of a variety of foods (because breast milk's taste changes, depending on what mom eats).

- Less food allergy (if nursed six or more months).

- Better antibody response to vaccinations.

- Decreased risk of Crohn's disease and ulcerative colitis (diseases that cause inflammation in the lower GI tract leading to chronic diarrhea).

- Reduced risk of diabetes.

- Reduced risk of juvenile rheumatoid arthritis.

- Lower cholesterol counts in adulthood.

- Less constipation.

- Breast milk's composition changes over time to suit baby's nutritional requirements.

- Breastfed babies are hospitalized ten times less often in the first year than formula-fed babies.

- Breastfeeding is prime bonding time for mother and child.

- Breastfed babies are leaner at one year than formula-fed babies, and are less likely to be obese later on.

For Mom

- Breastfed babies have much less offensive-smelling stool, which makes diaper changes a less-offensive chore.

- A mom who nurses for at least six months reduces her risk of breast, ovarian, cervical, and endometrial cancers.

- Exclusive nursing burns between 500 and 1,500 calories a day—a great aid to postpartum weight loss!

- Nursing causes mom's body to produce endorphins and other chemicals that relax her and promote mother-baby bonding.

- Exclusive nursing delays the return of fertility—although it shouldn't be your only form of birth control!

- Breast milk is always free, always heated to the right temperature, and always available. Simply by doing what comes naturally, you'll save thousands of dollars you would have spent on formula, bottles, nipples, and the other things you would need for bottle-feeding.

- You can nurse lying down, even sleeping. If you keep your baby near your bed at night, you can move the baby next to you, latch him on, and drift back to sleep. (If you are very overweight or obese, this may not be a good idea for you—the risk of the baby being smothered is greater. Also, use common sense when nursing lying down: keep heavy covers away from baby, and don't nurse this way with your baby wedged between you and the back of a couch.)

- Breastfeeding helps shrink the uterus faster postpartum.

While even a few weeks' worth of breastfeeding is better than none, it appears that the ideal is for the baby to get only breast milk for the first six months, and after that, to continue to nurse as a supplement to his diet until at least two years of age. This is from the World Health Organization's and American Academy of Pediatricians' recommendations. There is no nutritional advantage to giving your baby solids before six months of age, and introducing solids too soon can predispose your child to food sensitivities.

If you do bottle-feed, do *not* give your baby juice, soda, or sweetened beverages in her bottle. This introduces extra calories and sugars your baby doesn't need and promotes tooth decay. Do not give cow's milk to a baby under one-year-old.

Some women return to work in the first weeks or months of their baby's life. Many choose to switch to formula at that point, but you can choose instead to pump milk and continue giving your baby all of breast milk's benefits. Talk to a lactation consultant about this if you are interested.

YOUR CHILD'S EARLIEST SOLID FOODS: SIX TO EIGHT MONTHS

It's easy to get excited about introducing solids to your baby, especially when he seems so interested in grabbing at your spoon while you try to put food in your own mouth, or when you're hoping to fill him up enough to get him to sleep through the night. But for prevention of food allergies and for overall best health of your baby, the World Health Organization recommends not introducing solids to your baby until he is six months old.

Too-early feeding of solids can predispose a baby to overweight and obesity. Trying to feed solids too soon usually just ends up creating a colossal mess, since a baby younger than six months old has a strong tongue-thrust reflex that makes her push solid food out of her mouth. A baby under six months old is also at greater risk of gagging and choking than an older baby or child.

When that day finally comes to start feeding solids, parents can get a little nervous! Just take a deep breath and remember that when your baby starts on solids, he's learning a new skill. He is exercising muscles he hasn't used yet. Give him plenty of face-to-face interaction, smiles, and praise as he works on this new ability.

Don't give your baby refined grain foods like O-shaped cereal or crackers as her first food. Even though she might like these foods, they aren't nutrient dense. They contain a lot of sugars and/or refined carbohydrates, and will "set" her taste buds to a preference for bland and sweet foods.

Other foods to avoid before the age of twelve months are fish, shellfish, nuts, nut butters, seeds, citrus fruits, juices, egg whites, chili peppers, corn, soy, chocolate, honey, cow's milk, sugar, salt, soft cheeses, blue cheese, and anything small, hard, and easy to choke on.

Instead, try these first foods:

- Baby brown rice cereal or baby oatmeal mixed with breast milk or formula: Add enough liquid to thin the cereal to an almost liquid consistency. (You can make your own brown rice cereal by grinding uncooked brown rice in a food mill.) As your baby tries new fruits and vegetables, these can be mixed into brown rice cereal as well.

- Avocado: Just take a ripe avo, scoop it out, and mash it up. This can be thinned with breast milk or formula, or thickened with rice cereal for older babies.

- Portions of the family's meal, less spiced, pureed or otherwise processed (a hand-held baby food mill works great for this purpose).

- Carrots: Steam until soft, then mash.

- Banana: Mash in a bowl or run through a food mill. The mash can be thickened or thinned as above.

- Pears: If very soft and ripe, just peel and mash, or run through a food mill. If not soft, peel, cut into chunks, and steam until tender, then mash or mill.

Baby's Food Doesn't Have to Be Bland!

There's no need to make baby's first foods spiceless and bland. Believe it or not, studies show that when nursing mothers eat more garlic—which infuses breast milk with a garlicky taste—their infants nurse better! In some cultures, parents commonly feed babies with food rich in spices and herbs, helping to expand their tastes and improve their acceptance of more variety. Many herbs and spices also have medicinal value—for example, cinnamon helps keep blood sugar in healthy limits, ginger helps soothe upset tummies, and curry is loaded with natural antioxidants and anti-inflammatory compounds.

You can add cinnamon to cooked carrots or applesauce; ginger to cooked carrots or mashed bananas; curry powder to cooked, pureed chicken or vegetables; or cumin or sage to steamed vegetables. There is never any need to add salt to a baby's food, however.

- Winter squash (acorn, butternut, Hubbard): Cut in half, scoop out seeds, place facedown on a baking pan that has been filled inch-deep with water and cook at 400 degrees until soft. Or peel, scoop out seeds, cut into chunks, and boil until tender. Puree cooked squash and thin or thicken as needed.

- Sweet potato: Bake and scoop out of skin, or peel, cut up, and boil, then mash or puree.

- Ripe mango: Mash into a puree.

- Applesauce: Homemade or store-bought will do! The sauce can be mixed with rice cereal or oatmeal.

- Thoroughly pureed cooked meats, such as chicken, can be offered once the child is eating vegetables and fruits. Try mixing pureed meat with yam, carrot, or squash puree.

Most babies can hold and chew small chunks of soft foods by their first birthday. Teething can be addressed by giving a baby lightly steamed vegetable sticks or peeled raw fruit to chew on; chilling these foods helps even more.

Don't leave a baby alone to eat. Always be nearby to deal with choking emergencies.

MOVING ON: EIGHT MONTHS TO TWO AND A HALF YEARS

Some foods are best reserved for babies eight months of age or older. As your baby becomes a toddler, keep these restrictions in mind:

- After eight months of age, you can add egg yolk (not whites, which should not be introduced until after age one, as this helps prevent allergy to eggs—a very common food allergy).

- Avoid citrus fruit, honey, peanut butter, and products made from wheat until baby's first birthday.

- After age one, you can introduce plain, full-fat, live-culture yogurt. A child that doesn't taste the sweetened, fruity brands of yogurt will enjoy the sour tang of the real thing far more. You can always add a dash of maple syrup or fruit puree to add sweetness.

- Avoid introducing low-fat milk before the age of twenty-four months.

- If allergies run in your family, it may be best to continue to avoid common allergens such as nuts, egg whites, fish, and shellfish through to thirty-six months. Continue to avoid whole nuts until five years of age. When giving a new food, give only that food at the meal in which it's being introduced; that way, you can see clearly whether your baby reacts to it or not. When first introducing a new food, wait about three days before introducing another new food. This helps target any source of food allergies.

DESIGNING YOUR FAMILY'S MEALS

I've come up with a very simple way to design your family's meals—a way that allows even the youngest child to participate.

Here's how to get started. Sit down with your children and explain: "Now that we are all shifting to a healthier way of eating and getting lots of exercise together, it's time for us to work together more on family dinners and to eat together most nights of the week. This will be a new tradition in our family, and it's going to give us lots of great time together to talk and listen to each other. The first thing we're going to do is create a menu for this coming week, and I need your help."

Ask the children what their favorite meals are. If your children are like most children, they'll ask for cereal, bagels, or pastry for breakfasts, and PB & J, macaroni and cheese, pasta, chicken nuggets, burgers, hot dogs, pizza, or grilled cheese for lunches and dinners. Snacks will probably be things like chips, crackers, and sweets, or perhaps yogurt or string cheese will make the list.

Then, try to construct a menu that contains healthy versions of the meals they love. The general "layout" of such a menu can be broken down in very simple terms for your children.

Here's a *teachable moment*. Tell the children that each meal and snack needs to contain:

- A "growing food"—some protein from meat, eggs, beans, nuts, nut butters, cheese, or yogurt

- An "energy food"—some carbohydrates from whole grains like whole-wheat bread, tortillas, or crackers, brown rice, or corn

- A "vitamin and mineral food"—some fruit or vegetables

Creative parents can have fun coming up with their own terms that resonate with their children. See the sample meal plan on page 78.

Then, create your shopping list (you can use the version in this book on page 83, or create your own). Depending on the ages of your children, you can have them write their own lists, or you can write the lists for them to help them learn their letters and words.

Once you have your list, let the children help you figure out which meals you'll prepare for family dinners, and which they will have for breakfasts and lunches that week. Then, do your shopping.

Let the children know you expect them to participate with preparing family meals. Younger children will be able to help with spreading, mixing, pouring, and measuring, and as they grow older they can begin to help cut and even to do some of the cooking at the stove or oven.

The table on page 80 gives a few of children's favorite foods and some alternatives you can offer. A lot of these ideas involve mixing finely chopped or pureed vegetables into foods to boost their food value; if you think your child will turn up his nose at even the *idea* that a vegetable might be hidden in there, you may want to put him on table-setting duty or some other task while you slip in those secret ingredients!

SHOPPING SUCCESS

The Fit Family Food Plan revolves around *whole foods*, which may change the way you shop. The idea here is to keep certain whole-food staples in your fridge and pantry, and to turn to these foods instead of going out to eat a high-calorie meal or heating up some kind of boxed, prepared meal from your freezer.

Shop the periphery of your market—meaning, hit the produce, meat, seafood, and dairy sections, with a minimum of trips down the aisles where highly processed foods lurk, just waiting to capture your interest (and if you're shopping with a child, to potentially cause screaming tantrums when you refuse to buy them).

In the table on the following page are some ideas for foods to combine in your Fit Family Plan; you can use this as a grocery list, highlighting items you wish to buy. When possible, buy fruits and vegetables fresh when they are in season; if you can't do so, buy frozen versions.

Meal Plan for Fit Families

Try to stick with this nutritional plan Monday through Friday. Reward yourself over the weekend with whatever you're craving—but keep portion sizes small when you indulge in those "forbidden foods." In the Appendix, you'll find plenty of additional recipes to help you to create delicious meals for your family.

Water is always the best choice for a beverage!

Fit Family Breakfast

One protein food (growing food)

+ One vegetable or fruit (vitamin and mineral food)

+ One carbohydrate-rich food (energy food)

Examples:

• Oatmeal with non-fat milk and a cup of sliced fruit

• One or two slices of whole-grain bread or a whole-grain English muffin with peanut butter and honey, with a glass of orange juice or a few orange slices

• Egg burrito made with one scrambled egg, a tablespoon of grated cheese, and a tablespoon of salsa (add avocado if your child likes it); if the child doesn't like salsa, substitute fruit or vegetable juice

Snack

One fruit or vegetable (vitamin and mineral food)

+ protein or carbohydrate for kids with big appetites (growing food or energy food)

Examples:

• Apple slices with a few small cubes of cheddar cheese

• Celery sticks with nut butter and raisins

• Crackers with nut butter or cheese, and sliced berries or apples

• Plain yogurt with a tablespoon of granola and fresh fruit mixed in

• Grapes, orange, berries, apple, banana, or other fruit

• Raw veggie sticks (such as carrots) with Ranch dip

Lunch

One protein food (growing food)

+ One vegetable or fruit (vitamin and mineral food)

+ One carbohydrate-rich food (energy food)

Examples:

- Turkey sandwich made with tomato, light mayonnaise, and lettuce on whole-grain bread, plus a handful of grapes
- Fun whole-grain pasta shapes tossed with marinara sauce and finely chopped spinach or other vegetable with a sprinkling of Parmesan cheese
- Cheese and chicken quesadilla made with a whole-grain tortilla folded in half, plus apple slices

Snack

Same as mid-morning snack

Dinner

One protein food (growing food)

+ One vegetable or fruit (vitamin and mineral food)

+ One carbohydrate-rich food (energy food)

Examples:

- Grilled chicken breast*, rice, broccoli
- Baked salmon, potatoes, zucchini
- Refried beans with cheese melted on top, baked tortilla chips, apple slices

Be sure to check out the recipes in the back of the book for lots of Keeling-kid-tested, fun recipes that we enjoy preparing for our family dinners.

*We love our George Foreman Grill for preparing chicken, fish, vegetables—even fruits, which can be a delicious treat when grilled and served with vanilla yogurt or ice cream. These small indoor grills are very inexpensive compared to traditional outdoor grills, and they clean up far more easily.

HEALTHFUL ALTERNATIVES TO FAVORITE "KID FOODS"

KID FOOD: PB & J ON WHITE BREAD

Healthy homemade alternatives: Peanut butter or almond butter, and sugar-free fruit preserves or sliced fresh fruit, drizzled with honey on whole-grain bread

Teachable moment: "Whole grains have more vitamins and fiber, which help us have more energy and poop easier (!). This jam has no added sugar—it's just fruit, and fruit is loaded with vitamins that help you stay healthy and give you plenty of energy."

KID FOOD: MACARONI AND CHEESE

Healthy homemade alternatives: Use an organic mix made with whole-grain pasta. In the last minute of cooking the pasta, drop in a couple of handfuls of grated zucchini, peas, small florets of broccoli, very finely chopped spinach, or another vegetable your children will eat, or add pureed cooked butternut squash to the cheese sauce mixture before mixing into pasta. I like to also stir some diced chicken, turkey, soft tofu, or canned chunk-light tuna into the mac and cheese. Use organic plain yogurt instead of milk to make the cheese sauce.

Teachable moment: "Organic food is grown or made without chemicals that can be bad for your body. We add vegetables because they have so many vitamins and minerals your body needs, and we add chicken, turkey, tuna, or tofu for protein—the part of the food that helps you grow. Yogurt is actually milk from a cow that has special 'friendly' bacteria added to give it that sweet tangy taste and nice thickness—and those bacteria are good for your tummy!"

KID FOOD: FROZEN FRIED CHICKEN NUGGETS

Healthy homemade alternatives: Dip chicken tenders in 1 cup crushed corn flakes mixed with 1 cup bread crumbs, 2 tbsp. brown sugar, 1 tsp. salt, $1/2$ tsp. pepper, and $1/2$ tsp. allspice. Drizzle 3 tbsp. olive, canola, or peanut oil over the mixture and mix up with your hands to combine oil with crumbs completely. Cut chicken tenders into 2-inch strips, coat them with $1/3$ cup flour, then dip into 2 beaten eggs. Then press the chicken into the crumb mixture to coat. Arrange chicken on a non-stick baking sheet and cook for 15 minutes—they should become crisp and brown.

Teachable moment: "When a food is fried, it isn't as healthy for your body. When you get the food already made from the grocery store, it can have a lot more unhealthy ingredients in it—so we are going to make it ourselves, and we get to decide what we put in there . . . we are going to use eggs and corn flakes, which we sometimes eat for breakfast . . . and healthy oil, which your body needs to grow and heal."

KID FOOD: TAKEOUT OR DELIVERY PIZZA

Healthy homemade alternatives: Make your own, either using a pre-made refrigerated crust from the store or following a recipe to make your own (this takes a bit more time than many families have in the evening). You might even try using pitas or flatbreads. Spread them with an organic marinara sauce, and stir in a little extra minced garlic, grated zucchini, finely chopped tomatoes or onions, or thinly shredded spinach. Sprinkle on only as much grated mozzarella as you need to cover the sauce. Sprinkle on sliced olives, red peppers, or other veggies your kids like. If your family likes meat on its pizza, try a small amount of turkey sausage, white meat chicken, or turkey meatballs sliced in quarters. Bake for about 10 minutes in a 400°F oven if using pitas or flatbreads, or at 450°F if you are using a refrigerated or homemade crust, until cheese is bubbly and beginning to brown.

Teachable moment: "Pizza from the pizza shop can be very heavy, greasy and salty, so we are going to make a healthier version. Let's choose some vegetables we can chop up real small so that they blend into that yummy red sauce."

KID FOOD: BURGERS OR HOT DOGS AND FRENCH FRIES

Healthy homemade alternatives: Try replacing standard burgers with turkey burgers or salmon burgers. Use whole-grain buns. For the fries, try oven-baked potato chips. Thinly slice russet potatoes with a knife, mandoline, or food processor; spray with spray oil or lightly brush with olive oil; bake at 375°F until lightly browned; remove from oven and sprinkle with sea salt.

Teachable moment: "Turkey and fish are great growing foods, and are better for our bodies than regular hamburgers. You can still have the toppings you love. French fries are very unhealthy because of all the oil they contain and because they are fried. We're going to bake potato chips in the oven instead."

KID FOOD: WHITE PASTA WITH BUTTER AND PARMESAN CHEESE

Healthy homemade alternatives: Many stores now sell alternatives to white-flour pasta, including whole-wheat pasta and pasta made from other grains like rice. Try other types of noodles, like Japanese soba noodles (made with buckwheat flour) tossed with peanut sauce. If you do serve white pasta, find a tomato-based sauce your children will eat and stir in some very finely chopped greens or other vegetables. Roasted eggplant, garlic, and zucchini can be pureed and stirred into red sauce. If red sauce is out of the question, toss pasta with half olive oil and half butter instead of butter alone, or try one of the "buttery spreads" now sold that are more healthful than butter. Use a high-quality Parmesan cheese, as this will require using less of it to get the taste the kids love. Try to agree with the kids about one vegetable to add. Add a source of protein (sliced chicken or turkey sausage or ground turkey or chicken cooked up and added to the sauce).

Teachable moment: "All over the world, people eat different kinds of noodles. They make them from wheat, or rice, or another grain called buckwheat, and they use many different kinds of sauce. We're going to play around with some of these different tastes, because the sauces and different grains all have different vitamins and minerals your body needs."

KID FOOD: FAVORITE SNACKS LIKE CHIPS, CRACKERS, AND SWEETS

Healthy homemade alternatives: Tree nuts like almonds and cashews make wonderful snacks. Buy them dry-roasted, or buy them raw and roast them yourself in the oven—just toss with a little oil (about 1 tsp. per cup of nuts) and spread them evenly on a baking pan. Bake at 350°F, stirring occasionally, for 5 to 10 minutes—be sure not to let them burn. Sprinkle on a bit of salt when they come out; some kids love them generously sprinkled with cinnamon sugar. Keep nuts in the freezer if you won't be eating them within a week or so. For the ideal snack, pair a "growing food" (protein-rich food) with a vegetable or fruit: whole-grain crackers with nut butter and fresh fruit; celery and carrot sticks with light cream cheese; yogurt with fruit and granola; apple slices with almond butter or small cubes of sharp cheddar cheese.

Teachable moment: "When snack time comes around, we want to send lots of good vitamins, minerals, fats, and protein down into your tummy, and so we need to choose foods that supply all these things to keep you strong and help you think, jump, dance, and grow! Crackers and chips and sweets don't do that too well—they might taste good going in, but they leave your muscles hungry and you'll end up feeling yucky!"

KID FOOD: SWEET DESSERTS

Healthy homemade alternatives: It's fine to indulge sometimes in cake, candy, or cookies, but try to teach your kids that there are healthier alternatives that are just as delicious. Cut-up fresh fruit or frozen berries with a dollop of vanilla yogurt can be a very satisfying finish to a family meal. Cut fruit into fun shapes and let the kids eat it with toothpicks.

Seek out healthy cookie recipes (or pre-made cookies) that use oatmeal, dried fruits, nuts, whole-grain flour, and little processed sugar. On a special night, enjoy with a small scoop of high-quality ice cream. (It's so rich and delicious that you don't need to eat as much; encourage your child to eat it slowly and savor each bite by handing out small spoons.) High-quality chocolate is another fun choice—hand out a small serving to each family member to savor slowly—and cocoa is known to contain antioxidants that are good for your family's health!

Teachable moment: "Sweets are 'sometime foods,' but we can eat fruit any time—and fruit is so sweet and delicious! When we do have a sweet treat, it's really fun to eat it slowly and enjoy it with all our senses . . . smell it, look at it, taste it all over your tongue!"

SAMPLE WHOLE-FOODS SHOPPING LIST

PROTEIN

Canned chunk-light tuna in water

Chicken breasts

Cod

Eggs

Flank steak

Ground beef (85% lean) or ground turkey

Halibut

Peanut butter or almond butter

Salmon

Snapper

Turkey

CARBOHYDRATES

Corn

Corn tortillas

Lentils

Oatmeal (instant or slow-cooked)

Pasta (whole-grain when possible)

Potatoes

Rice (brown or white)

Whole-grain cereals (low in sugar)

Whole-grain muffins or bagels

Whole-grain or sourdough bread

Yams

VEGETABLES

Asparagus

Broccoli

Cabbage

Carrots

Cauliflower

Celery

Chard

Collard greens

Cucumber

Green beans

Mushrooms

Onions

Romaine lettuce

Spinach

Tomatoes

Zucchini

DAIRY

Cottage cheese

Goat cheese (a good substitute for cream cheese or to crumble into salads)

Milk (low-fat or fat-free)

Parmesan cheese

Plain yogurt

Sharp cheddar cheese

FRUITS

Apples

Bananas

Blueberries

Cantaloupe

Grapefruit

Grapes

Kiwi

Orange juice

Oranges

Peaches

Pineapple

Plums

Raisins*

Raspberries

Strawberries

Watermelon

* Eat dried fruits like raisins in moderation, as they have high-caloric density and sugar content.

CONDIMENTS

Honey	Salad dressing (low-fat)
Mayonnaise (non-fat)	Salsa
Mustard	Vinegars

SNACKS

Baby carrots	Pretzels/crackers
Fruit smoothie	Single-serving yogurt or cottage cheese
Nutrition bars	String cheese
Nuts	Trail mix

UNLIMITED!

Balsamic vinegar	Pepper
Fresh basil	Salsa
Garlic	WATER!

CHAPTER 5

Fitness-Loving Kids
Fitness for School-Aged Children and Their Parents

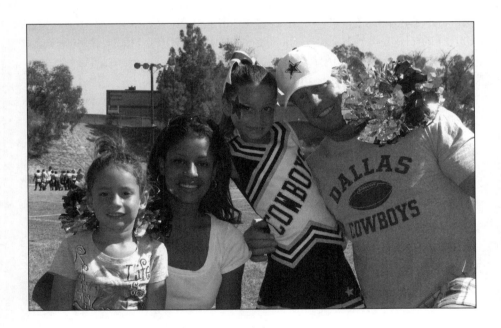

As many headlines have screamed about obesity being as dangerous as smoking and about how the fattening of America threatens to destroy the U.S. health-care system, many researchers have gone about proving that you can be overweight or obese and *fit*—and that being fit, from regular exercise, has the same health benefits whether you move into a more ideal weight category or not.

For both parents and children, being physically fit leads to more energy, better mood, better sleep at night, a stronger body more resistant to injury, longer life, and less disease. Being fit, for example, substantially reduces your risk of cardiovascular disease, colon cancer, diabetes, and high blood pressure. All these changes will come with improved physical fitness, *no matter what your BMI.*

Unfortunately, most modern Americans are *not* physically fit. According to the Centers for Disease Control and Prevention (CDC), about 60 percent of us do not get the recommended amount of physical activity. And while children are more likely to be physically active than adults, they seem to be having an increasingly hard time maintaining an active life once they reach their 'tween and teen years.

Researchers in San Diego, California did a study involving 1,032 children, ages nine to fifteen, who wore small activity monitors to track their daily exercise habits between the years 2000 and 2006. The study was published in the *Journal of the American Medical Association* (*JAMA*). On average, on weekdays, the nine-year-old children did about 179.2 minutes (about three hours) of moderate to vigorous physical activity per day; by the time this same group was fifteen, they were doing only 43.1 minutes per day on average. Another way of looking at this data: while 90 percent of nine-year-olds get a couple of hours of exercise on most days, *fewer than 3 percent of fifteen-year-olds get this amount of exercise.* Rising prevalence of obesity reflects this trend.

Families who want to buck this trend face many obstacles, including reduced P.E. time for children in school, more homework, more "screen time," and lack of safe places to go to be active. Although many children end up involved in sports programs that help keep them active on some days, it's important for parents not to rely on these programs as the child's only source of physical activity and to emphasize that for elementary-aged children, team sports are about fun, not about winning.

The Fit Family Plan is all about creating healthy exercise habits from the very start so that kids can keep that momentum going for a lifetime. My intention in this chapter is to offer you so many great, inexpensive, fun ideas for getting and staying fit with your children that you won't even consider not going for it!

ACTIVE, FIT KIDS FROM PRESCHOOL AGE FORWARD

If you have or have ever had a one- to two-and-a-half-year-old, you know that their being physically active is a given. As soon as a child this age finds his or her legs and starts scooting, walking, and running, parents tend to run themselves ragged trying to keep up! The main goal of any parent who has a child this age is to keep him safe as he explores and plays. As he does this, encourage him and expect him to get lots of bumps and bruises—that's just part of learning to get around.

You will probably still find yourself carrying a child this age quite often. The sling carriers mentioned in Chapter 6 are great for this age group, as they can be used to carry even a big toddler on one hip or piggy-back (on the back of the hips) without hampering the adult's alignment.

A jogging stroller can help you stay active during this time. Once your child is near or at age three, however, it may be time to give that stroller or jogger away to someone with a younger child.

According to the American Academy of Pediatrics, it's okay to use a stroller while your child is an infant or toddler, but by the time he or she is three, it's time to let the child walk. Busy parents often find that letting a preschooler out of the stroller to walk alongside them takes more time than they have. Some preschoolers love to run off on their own, and an attempt to run an errand can turn into a game of tag that's great fun for the child, but a major headache for the time-pressed adult.

Although it can be difficult, try to embrace the fundamental truth that children need to move around and explore their environments. If they get in the habit of sitting in a stroller too often, watching the world go by in a passive manner, they may begin heading toward a sedentary lifestyle, and face increased risk of obesity.

HOW MUCH ACTIVITY DOES YOUR CHILD NEED
TO BE HEALTHY?

Although you can find recommendations for children that are similar to those for adults—for example, sixty minutes per day of moderate to vigorous physical activity—experts agree that creating hard-and-fast guidelines for children's optimal physical activity is difficult.

Children don't exercise like adults. They do it in fits and starts, stopping and starting often, and at greatly varying levels of intensity. Trying to apply guidelines to this kind of exercise will likely be impossible. And there's no need to try; any young child, given proper space and time, will be physically active. It's in their makeup to jump, run, and actively play. They may be even more likely to do so when they have peers around to jump, run, and play with. It follows that organizing playdates with other moms can help keep all of you active. Children will also follow your lead as you become more active.

Allow children who are playing together to organize and create their own games. This is an important aspect of development that helps children learn cooperation and collaboration.

Get creative about ways to be active, even at home. Some families have tried:

- A mini-tramp or trampoline indoors

- Ropes for climbing and swinging

- A swing hung from a backyard tree

- A Thera-ball for rolling on and playing with inside the house

- Dance videos that children can follow

- Removing or moving some furniture to create more open space inside the home to invite more physical play

CARDIOVASCULAR CONDITIONING: MYTHS AND REALITIES

Many people are under the impression that you need to do a certain amount of cardio—for example, walking, running, swimming, or cycling—*plus* a certain amount of strength training to get and stay fit. When working out effectively seems to entail at least an hour, four or five times a week (say, thirty to forty-five minutes of cardio, plus strengthening and stretching work), it can seem just plain out of the question.

The truth is that cardiovascular training and strength training can be done separately, but that they can also be combined very effectively. Time-efficient workouts include both of these elements—raising heart rate by incorporating lots of full-body strengthening moves like squats and lunges, and some intervals of moderate- to high-intensity cardio. The workouts supplied in this book will fulfill your body's needs for both cardio and strengthening. When and if you can add walking, cycling, running, dancing, swimming, or any other cardio to these workouts, go for it—you'll reap even more benefits! But if you go from being a couch potato to doing one of these workouts on most days of the week, your fitness will improve, you'll get stronger both muscularly and "cardiovascularly," and your energy and sleep quality will improve.

If you're wanting to drop a significant amount of weight, you will probably want to include extra cardio elements on most days so that you total an hour of time with your heart rate up between 65 and 85 percent of your age-predicted maximum (see the inset on the following page to find your target heart rate). You may find that your heart rate stays within that range while doing the workouts supplied in this book—and if this is the case, you can definitely count the time spent there toward your daily hour of cardio.

This, when done along with keeping calorie intake in check with a whole-foods diet, has proved to be the only way to drop weight and keep it off.

The workouts supplied in this book are actually a form of *interval training*. Interval training entails getting heart rate up fairly high—into moderately high or high levels for your age—and keeping it there for a brief period, maybe thirty seconds to a minute. Then, you get a brief rest, just long enough to feel your heart rate drop back down toward normal, before starting your next exercise. Intervals are a great training tool to improve cardiovascular fitness and burn lots of calories. If you can get heart rate up high in your intervals, you'll continue to burn extra calories in the hours following as your metabolism stays high.

You can add extra intervals to all the workouts supplied here by inserting three to five one- to two-minute periods of running, stair climbing, trampoline jumping, energetic dancing, or hill walking. If you do this, keep your heart rate below your age-predicted maximum at all times, and keep moving as you recover from higher-intensity work.

As long as you are in good health and not pregnant, interval training should be safe for you. If you have any doubts about this, check with your doctor.

Your Training Heart Rate

220 Minus Age Equals Maximum Heart Rate

To get your Training Heart Rate (THR) in beats per minute, we're going to subtract your Resting Heart Rate (RHR) from your Maximum Heart Rate (MHR). Then, we're going to take a percentage of that—from 50 to 85 percent, depending on your fitness level—and add your RHR back in.

So, the formula looks like this:

$$MHR - RHR \times \text{intensity level} + RHR = THR$$

Confused? Don't worry. Here's further explanation.

The *intensity level* describes how hard you exercise as a percentage of your Maximum Heart Rate.

- If you are a beginner or have a low fitness level, your intensity level will be 50 to 60 percent.

- If you are of average fitness level, your intensity level will be 60 to 70 percent.

- If you are at a high fitness level, your intensity level will be 75 to 85 percent.

The Resting Heart Rate is the number of beats in one minute when you are at rest. You can check your RHR any time you are sitting or standing in a relaxed way. Average is between 80 and 100 beats.

Let's say you are thirty-years-old and you are of average fitness level. Your age-predicted MHR would be 190 beats per minute. You count your RHR and find it's 80 beats per minute. MHR minus RHR is 110. Multiply 110 by 60 percent and you get 66; multiply 110 by 70 percent and you get 77. Add your RHR back in: 66 plus 80 equals 146 and 77 plus 80 equals 157.

To do a 10-second pulse count, divide each of these answers by 6. That comes out to about 24 to 26 beats per ten seconds.

THE PLAYGROUND WORKOUT

One great place for a preschooler or elementary schooler to get exercise: your local playground. I can't tell you how many times I've seen children romping and playing at the playground where we bring our daughters, while their mothers or fathers sit on benches reading, talking on their cell phones, or chatting. Next time I see this, I hope to have a few copies of my book on hand . . . then, I can hand these folks a copy and say, "Hey—Mom [or Dad]—check out Chapter 5. You're missing a prime opportunity to get a workout in for yourself while your child plays on the playground!"

How? With my mom-tested, twenty-minute playground workout! This workout was born when my wife complained of not being able to fit an extra one or two workouts per week into her busy schedule caring for our daughters. The playground workout solved her problem—and she really enjoys it. It sets a great example for the kids, who notice she's exercising even as they play. If the child asks what you're up to, go ahead and tell him that you are exercising to get stronger, feel better, and have more energy— there's your *teachable moment*. They might even join in for a couple of sets!

If you're looking for a good warm-up, you might suggest a game of tag to your child. You'll get your heart pumping and raise your metabolism, and the kids love it. Be careful: those jungle gyms are made for the little ones. (In other words: watch your head.)

This workout focuses on large-muscle-group upper and lower body resistance exercises. When done back-to-back, without long rests, these exercises will get your heart rate up and keep it there, so you'll be doing both resistance training and cardio. A game of tag to warm up and a few sprints at the end (more on this later) will round out the cardiovascular portion of your workout.

I have listed these exercises in an order that makes sense based on which piece of playground equipment is used in each exercise, but they can be done in any order as you follow your little one around the playground.

Use this workout any time you are at the playground, but to build strength and endurance, try to do it at least twice a week. As you gain strength, add repetitions and sets to the series. For example, unless otherwise stated in the individual exercises, start out with ten repetitions; then, gradually increase to fifteen repetitions; then add a second set of ten to fifteen repetitions; and so on.

MONKEY BAR OR SWING-SET LEG LIFTS

For the abs.

STARTING POSITION: Reach up with both hands to hang from a bar along the monkey bars or the top rail of a swing set.

ACTION: Beginners can then lift one knee at a time toward the chest; more advanced exercisers can lift both knees at once. Keep the leg(s) bent at 90 degrees at the knee as you lift them. You can vary this by adding a twist, bringing the knees toward one or the other shoulder, alternating.

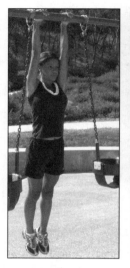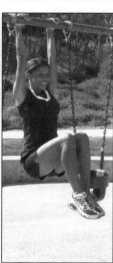

MONKEY BAR PULL-UPS

For the lats (the muscles that attach the upper arms to the spine), upper back, and biceps.

STARTING POSITION: Hang from both hands from a low bar on the jungle gym—about 3$\frac{1}{2}$ to 4 feet from the ground. Walk your feet out so that your hips are just below the bar and your legs slightly bent, with the soles of your feet flat on the ground.

ACTION: Pull your chest up toward the bar, letting the hips lift and the legs come toward straight. Almost touch your chest to the bar, then lower.

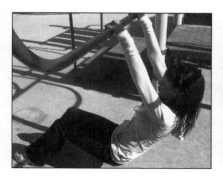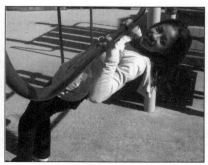

PARK BENCH PUSH-UPS

For the chest, triceps, and abs.

STARTING POSITION: Beginners can do this one with hands on the back of the bench; stronger moms or dads can put their hands on the edge of the seat of the bench. Get into a push-up position.

ACTION: Lower the chest down until the elbows are at a 90-degree angle, then straighten the arms. Give me 10 to 15! Remember to engage your abs —"zip" them up, lifting your belly inward and up as you do this exercise.

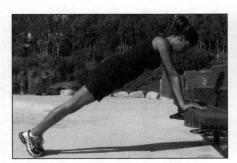
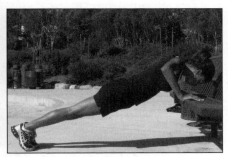

PARK BENCH MOUNTAIN CLIMBERS

For the legs, hips, butt, abs, and arms, and for cardiovascular conditioning.

STARTING POSITION: Place both palms on the seat of a bench.

ACTION: "Run" your legs behind you, switching the legs into lunges with alternate knees in front. Do 15 to 20 repetitions, with one rep being one lunge with right knee front and one lunge with left knee front.

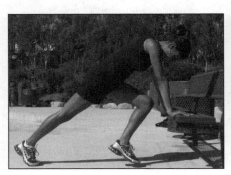
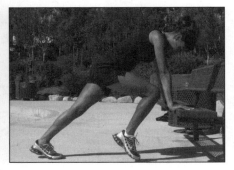

PARK BENCH TRI-DIP

For the triceps.

STARTING POSITION: Sit down on the edge of a bench, feet flat on the ground. Place the heels of both hands beside your hips, then shift your hips off the edge of the bench to hold your weight on your hands.

ACTION: Keep your shoulders pressed down away from your ears as you bend your elbows to lower your hips toward the ground, then press back to straight. The more you keep your knees bent, the easier this will be; as you get stronger, you can walk your feet farther away from the bench.

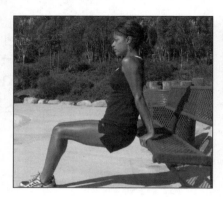 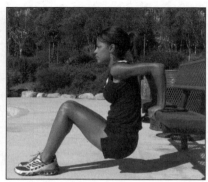

PARK BENCH AIR SQUATS

Strengthens and tones the entire lower body.

STARTING POSITION: Stand facing away from a park bench, close enough that you would sit down on its very edge if you squatted down and back far enough. Lift your arms directly overhead.

ACTION: Squat down until your bottom almost touches the bench, reaching your arms out in front of you, then return to standing, lifting the arms overhead again. Repeat 10 to 12 times.

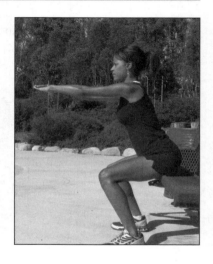

PARK BENCH SINGLE-LEG STEP-UPS

Strengthens and tones the entire lower body.

STARTING POSITION: Stand facing the park bench.

ACTION: Step onto its seat with one foot, reaching arms overhead. Exhale as you use the strength of the leg and hip to lift your body weight up onto the bench, bending both elbows and pulling them back behind you to work the upper back. Keep the other leg behind you slightly so that the foot points down to the spot on the ground from which you just stepped. Place hands on hips and descend back to starting position. Repeat 5 to 8 times on the same leg before switching sides.

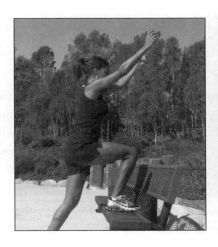 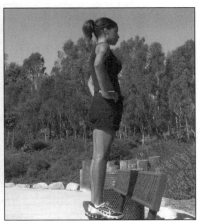

PARK BENCH SINGLE-LEG KICKBACK

For the hips and butt.

STARTING POSITION: Stand facing a park bench with a back. Lean forward and grasp the back of the bench with both hands. (See next page.)

ACTION: Bring your right knee up toward your chest as far as it will go, keeping the knee of the standing leg slightly bent. Then, extend that same leg out behind you until your head, torso, and leg are in a long line, parallel to the ground. Hold for two seconds, then return the knee to your chest. Repeat 12 to 15 times per side.

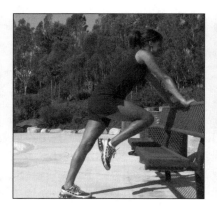 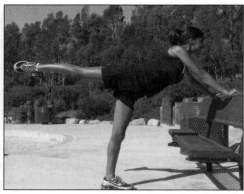

PARK BENCH SEATED AB CRUNCH

To strengthen your core.

STARTING POSITION: Sit on the edge of a park bench.

ACTION: Grip the bench's edge, then balance on your butt, lifting your knees up as high as you can toward your chest as you lean back to counterbalance. Exhale as your knees crunch in, then inhale as you extend your legs out straight and lean your upper body back a little more. Exhale as you crunch your knees in again.

At first, you may only be able to partially straighten your knees, and you may only lower them a small amount toward the ground. As you get stronger, you'll be able to almost do a complete layout, so that your heels almost touch the ground as you straighten your knees. Repeat this move 15 to 20 times.

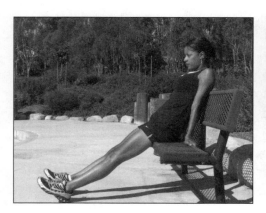 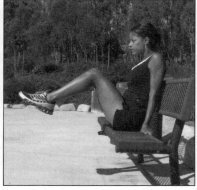

PARK BENCH LATERAL STEP-UP

Strengthens and tones the entire lower body.

STARTING POSITION: Stand with your left side toward the park bench.

ACTION: Step onto the bench's seat with your left foot, reaching your arms out to the sides. Exhale as you use the strength of the leg and hip to lift your body weight up onto the bench, swinging both arms around to your sides and overhead as you press your left knee straight. Tap your right toes next to your left foot before stepping softly back down with the right foot, following it with your left foot. After you descend back to starting position, repeat 5 to 8 times on the same leg before switching sides.

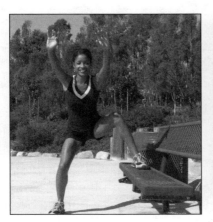 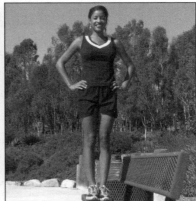

SWING SQUATS

For allover lower body conditioning.

STARTING POSITION: If your child loves to swing, you can keep exercising while you push him. Stand in your usual swing-pushing spot, with your feet at least shoulder-width apart. (See next page.)

ACTION: As you push the child, squat your hips down and back, keeping knees behind toes and heels on the ground. Keep your gaze forward and exaggerate the reach forward in your arms, then stand tall again as you wait for the child to swing back your way.

Variation: Step one foot wide to the side as you squat, then bring the feet together as you stand upright again; on the next push, lunge to the other side.

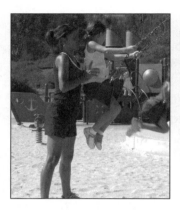 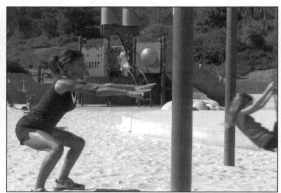

SWING PRESS FRONT LUNGE

More full lower body conditioning. Alternate swing squats with this exercise.

STARTING POSITION: Same as that for the swing squats in the exercise above.

ACTION: As you push the child in the swing, lunge forward onto one leg and drop the other knee toward the ground. Lunge so that the forward knee is at a 90-degree angle, with the whole foot on the ground. As you wait for the child to swing back toward you, push off the front foot and bring the feet together, then repeat on the next swing with the other foot in front. Repeat 10 to 20 times, alternating legs.

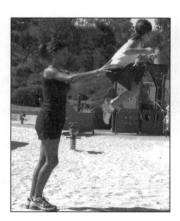 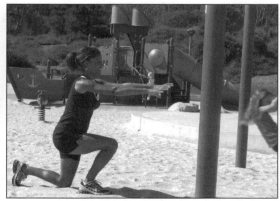

POLE SQUATS

More overall lower body conditioning. This is a good one for beginning exercisers.

STARTING POSITION: Hold on to one of the play structure's poles with one or both hands, feet set wide apart. (If you hold with one hand, put the other hand on your hip.)

ACTION: Squat the hips down and back, pulling back against the pole until your knees are at 90 degrees. Heels should stay on the ground throughout. Go slowly! Repeat this one 10 to 16 times.

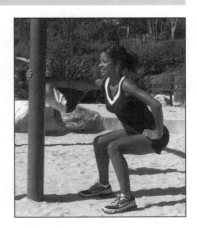

POLE PLIÉS

Works the inner thighs, backs of hips, and entire leg.

STARTING POSITION: Still holding on to the pole, spread your feet more than shoulder-width apart. Rotate your legs out from the hips, so that the toes and knees turn out by about 45 degrees. This one is much like the sumo squat on page 40, but works the inner thighs and back of the hips a bit more.

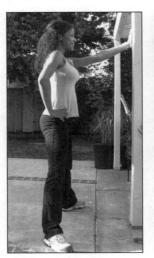
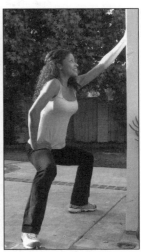

ACTION: Sink your hips straight down toward the ground, pressing knees out to the side as you descend. Keep heels on the ground. Return to starting position and repeat 10 to 12 times.

POLE UPPER BODY STRETCH

STARTING POSITION/ACTION: After finishing your last pole squat, sit into one more squat and pull back, holding tight to the pole to stretch your upper back and lats. Drop your chin toward your chest and hold for 30 to 60 seconds.

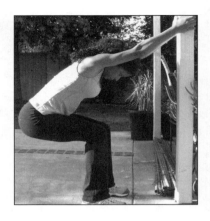

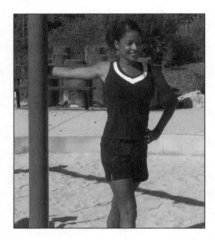

POLE CHEST STRETCH

STARTING POSITION/ACTION: Stand up and reach for the pole with one hand, grasping it at chest level. Turn away from that arm so that you feel a stretch in your chest on that side. Hold for 30 to 60 seconds, then switch sides.

POLE CALF STRETCH

Builds strength of calf and foot muscles.

STARTING POSITION: Bring the feet together, still holding on to the pole or to another sturdy part of the play structure.

ACTION: Rise on the balls of the feet, hold for a count of two, and lower. Repeat 15 to 20 times. For a greater challenge, place one foot around the ankle of the other foot and do one foot at a time.

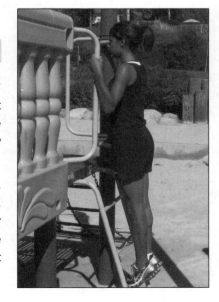

SPRINTS

We enjoy doing these as a family before we go home from the playground. It's actually Nikki's and my favorite part of the park workout!

We take the girls on a straightaway 50 to 100 yards long and do sprints one at a time (to defuse competition—the girls used to cry if we all ran together and they didn't win). Everybody does a countdown of "Five! Four! Three! Two! One!" and a parent takes off to set the pace and distance. We all cheer as the parent crosses the finish line, and then it's the next person's turn. Then, once we've had a chance to cheer everyone on past the finish line, we all jog back together to the starting line. We each do five or six sprints total.

The sprints usually bring a great *teachable moment:* When your child starts to sweat and breathe hard, explain to him or her that getting hot and sweating is good for the body. It means that the lungs are being expanded and the heart is being exercised to make both stronger and better able to move blood and oxygen around in the body. Let the child know that practicing these sprints will end up making her able to go faster and faster.

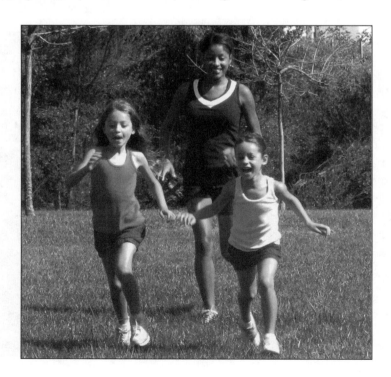

PLAYGROUND WORKOUT STRETCHES

Hold each of the following strectches for thirty to sixty seconds. Invite the kids to join you for these—they tend to think stretching is fun, and it's good for their physical development to try to imitate these positions. You can practice counting to thirty with the child as you hold the stretches, or sing a song that lasts about that long to measure the time.

HIP STRETCH

Cross one ankle over the other knee and sit back into a squat on the other leg. Reach both hands out front. In the image below, it's being done as a balance challenge as well as a stretch, but you can hold on to a pole or other object if you'd rather focus on the stretch alone.

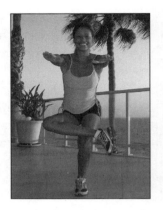

QUADRICEP/HIP FLEXOR STRETCH

Stand on one leg, reaching back for the other foot or ankle. Try to point the knee of the lifted leg down toward the ground, pressing the hip on the side of the lifted leg forward. You can use a park bench—either using its back for balance, or placing the lifted foot on the seat of the bench.

You can challenge your balance by not holding on to anything as you grasp your foot with the hand on that same side.

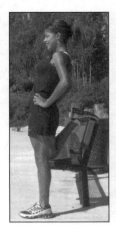
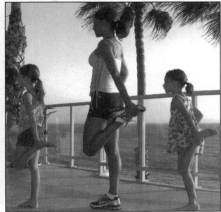

HAMSTRING STRETCH

Stand facing a bench, platform, or other high surface. Put one leg up onto that surface, flexing the foot so that the toes point back toward your face. Bend forward over the extended leg, reaching for the toes. Switch sides.

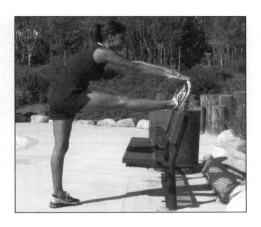

POLE UPPER BODY STRETCH

(For instructions, see page 100.)

POLE CHEST STRETCH

(For instructions, see page 100.)

YOGA FOR PARENTS AND KIDS

I got this series of yoga exercises from Melissa Lynn Block, a mom who is also a yoga and dance teacher. This series is great for a rainy-day activity at home, or as a way to energize *and* relax after or before a busy day. The names of the poses can change according to your family's own creative take on each exercise! Feel free to use music for these exercises—something with a beat that is not too distracting or overwhelming is best.

First, tell the children that in yoga, we breathe deep, and breathing is part of many of the movements. Have them practice taking deep, relaxed breaths before beginning this series. Unless it is otherwise stated, do each of these exercises facing your child or facing into a circle with your children.

SUN SALUTATION

Place your hands in a prayer position against your breastbone. Have everyone inhale, lifting hands up to the ceiling; then exhale, swan-diving out over their legs to hang forward, reaching toward the floor. (Keep the knees slightly bent.) Inhale, come halfway up, making a tabletop with your backs, then exhale back down to reach toward the floor again. Then inhale and reverse that swan-dive, spreading arms out to the side to stand straight up, fingertips reaching for the ceiling. Then, bring the hands back to prayer position in front of the heart. Repeat 3 to 5 times.

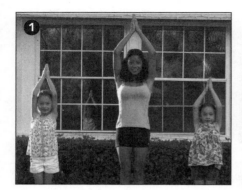

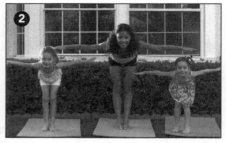

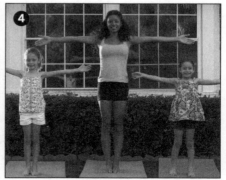

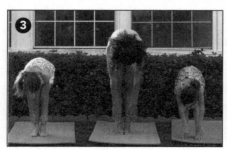

ANIMAL WALKS

Put your hands on the floor so that you're on both hands and both feet, with your hips up in the air. Have everyone walk around the room on all fours. You can take turns calling out different four-legged-animal names and changing the quality of the walks to match: dog, elephant, rhino, lizard, lion, and so on.

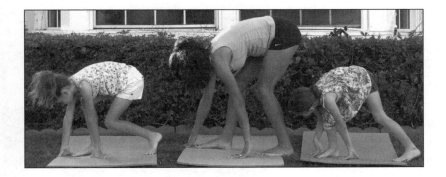

CRESCENT MOON

Stand up straight, facing your child or in a circle or a line with all your children. Reach one arm up high and curve your body so you're shaped like a crescent moon. Look up at the lifted hand, stretching longer with each inhalation. Try rising up on your tiptoes and back down. Repeat on the other side.

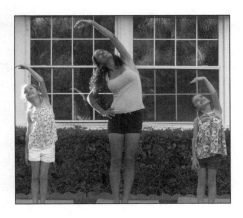

HALF MOON

If you want a big balance challenge, follow Crescent Moon with Half Moon: come back to standing up straight, then step out sideways onto the right foot, reaching the right hand toward the ground; lift the left foot up in the air, so your weight is only on your right hand and right foot as your left leg floats up toward the ceiling. Reach your left arm straight up toward the ceiling as well. Hold for a few breaths, floating upward with the inhalations, then change sides.

WIPING THE FLOOR

Stand with feet spread way out wide—farther than hip-width. Put both hands down on the floor, bending one knee and keeping the other leg more or less straight, then shift your weight over to the other side by bending the other knee and straightening the one that's

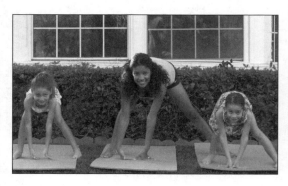

bent. Let the hands trail back and forth on the floor as if you're wiping it with both hands, breathing deeply. Do this slowly, 10 or so times.

BACKWARD LOOKING

Turn away from your children and have them turn away from you. Keep your legs spread wide and turn your feet to where they are parallel to each other. Clasp both hands behind your back and fold forward over your legs, keeping them slightly bent at your knees. Look back between your legs at the faces of your children, and let your clasped hands fall toward the back of your head to stretch your shoulders and chest. Hold for a few breaths.

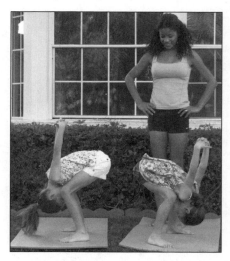

Then, add a twist: let your hands unclasp, and reach your right hand for your left ankle, reaching your left arm up toward the ceiling—keep looking at each other!—then, reverse by clasping your left hand to your right ankle and reaching your right arm up to the ceiling. When you've done this a few times, bend your knees even more, then roll your body back up to standing, slowly.

GOPHER

If you've ever seen a gopher trying to figure out whether it's safe for him to dart out of his hole, you'll know where this movement got its name. Stand in a circle facing each other. Roll your body down and bend your knees until your hands are on the floor. Let your head hang down. Make sure you have enough space in the middle of the circle before proceeding to dart yourself forward by walking out quickly onto your hands, until your body makes a plank shape. Look out in front of you. Then, walk your body back on your hands to stand on your feet, hanging forward over your slightly bent knees, head hanging forward, and roll back up to where you started. Your children can have fun making sounds as they dart forward. Can they think of other animals this movement reminds them of? Repeat 8 times.

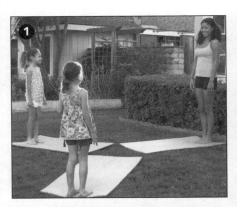

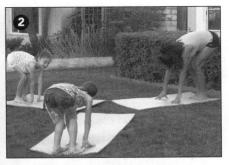

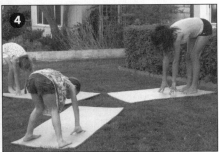

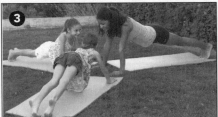

TREE

Stand on one leg and put the other foot against the thigh of the standing leg. Place hands in prayer position in front of your heart and balance for about half a minute on one leg, then switch sides.

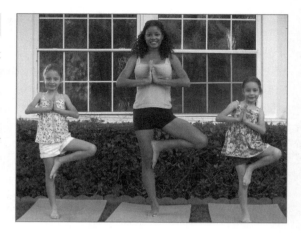

SNAKE

Get into a push-up position, head toward your children. Lower your body slowly to the floor on your belly. Come up onto your elbows or hands, shoulders away from ears, hips and legs and feet still on the floor, into a cobra position, inhaling; then, make a snake face by opening your mouth wide, sticking your tongue way out, and exhaling! Inhale again, then push yourself back into child's pose, where you sit back on your heels, legs folded, and fold your body over your thighs, forehead on the floor. Repeat 5 to 8 times. On the last repetition, stay in child's pose for a few breaths, then come up to your hands and knees.

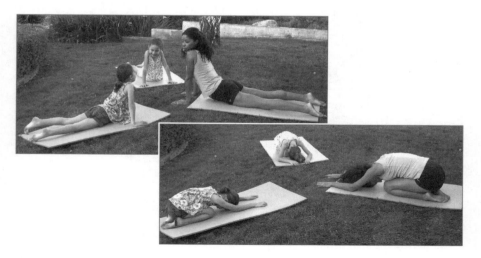

CAT/DOG

On all fours, inhale as you look up at the ceiling and stick your tailbone up toward the ceiling, dropping your belly and arching your back (dog pose). Think of a happy dog ready to play. Then, lift your belly and back toward

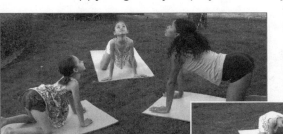

the ceiling as you drop your head and tail down (cat pose), thinking of a stretching cat getting up from his nap. Repeat 4 to 5 times.

BUTTERFLY BOUNCE

Sit with soles of feet together and bounce knees toward the floor, 12 to 20 times.

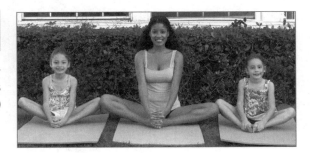

ROCKING THE BOAT

Sit on your bottom, legs up in the air and arms reaching past them or holding the backs of your knees so that you're balancing on your bottom—this is boat position. (See next page.) The more you bend your knees, the easier it will be to hold this position. Holding the backs of your knees, gently rock yourself backward, massaging out your spine against the floor (careful here if you have any neck problems—don't roll so far that you feel it in your neck). Return to balance in boat pose; then, gently fall forward so that the backs of your legs come to the floor, and fold your upper body forward over your legs. Then, sit back and lift your legs to come back into boat pose. Repeat all three poses (boat, rock back, fold forward) 5 times. You can play around with sound effects here—counting down from ten to "blastoff" in boat position, whooping "Whhhoooooooa!" as you roll back and into the forward bend, for example.

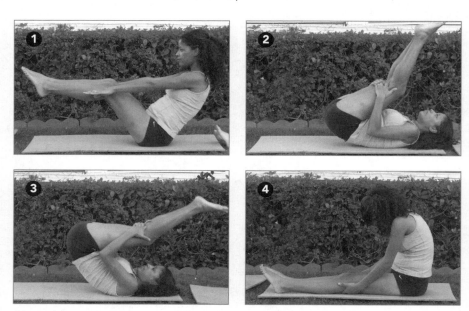

STARFISH

Lie on your back, arms and legs spread. Hug knees into chest, then reach right leg and left arm toward the ceiling as you reach left leg and right arm out along the floor; come back to the hugging knees position and reach left leg and right arm toward the ceiling as you reach right leg and left arm out along the floor. (If this is too hard for the children, have them simply hug their knees in, then open their body wide on the floor in the shape of a big starfish.) Repeat 10 times, then hug both knees in.

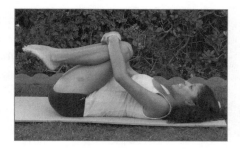

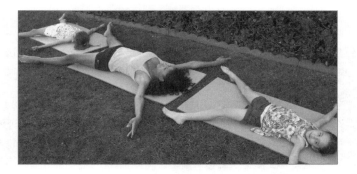

TWISTING

Send both knees to the left. Keep both shoulders on the ground and arms spread at shoulder level. Look right. Hold for a few breaths, then switch knees and gaze.

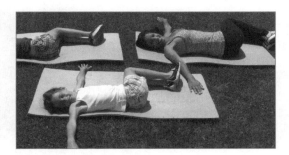

PEELING AND ROLLING

Lie on your back, feet on the floor near the hips, feet and knees hip-width apart. Begin "peeling" your back off the floor, starting at the very tip of your tailbone, lifting your hips off the floor, then your lower back, until you are holding your weight on your feet, upper back, and shoulders. (Head remains on the floor, neck

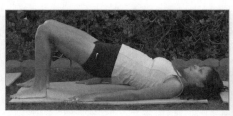

long.) Try lifting one leg at a time toward the ceiling for a more intense strengthening.

Then, reverse the peeling motion, rolling your back onto the floor from the top down. Repeat 6 to 8 times.

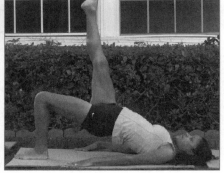

HIBERNATING BEAR

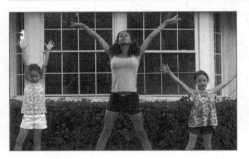

Stretch your body every which way like a bear about to go into his den for the winter. Then lie totally relaxed on your back. (Parents can cover their children with blankets to keep them warm as their bodies cool off.) Stay there for five to ten minutes.

If the kids get wiggly, try putting on some soothing music, or introduce a meditation like this one. Read it slowly, pausing between sentences to give the children a chance to visualize completely what you are saying:

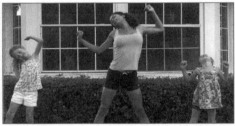

Imagine that you are a tree. Think of your roots reaching far, far down into the earth. Think of your leaves reaching up toward the sun. Feel the warm morning sun on your leaves. Feel drops of dew on your leaves. Feel your branches reaching out and growing. Trees breathe like we do. Feel yourself breathing like a tall tree, growing up toward the sun and down deep into the cool earth. Feel yourself full of calm energy. Does that energy have a color? Fill yourself from your toes to the crown of your head with that energy.

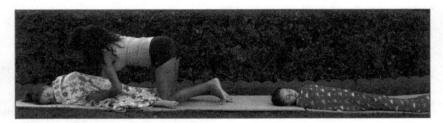

You can definitely come up with your own meditations. If the yoga turns out to be something you enjoy, check your local library for books on children's yoga. If you like yoga for yourself, keep in mind that yoga for children and yoga for adults are very different—but it's a great thing to explore for lifelong fitness and well-being.

FOR THE EXTREMELY BUSY: EXERCISE "SNACKS"

The CDC recommends that adults get thirty minutes per day of exercise, most days of the week—enough to burn about 210 calories. A study from Harvard University, however, found the lowest death rates in people who burned at least 300 calories per day doing some kind of exercise or physical activity.

If this sounds daunting to you, keep in mind that cutting these thirty-plus minutes per day into ten-minute chunks, or even five-minute chunks, doesn't reduce its health benefits. Do some squats and heel raises while brushing your teeth. Do some abdominal exercises while taking a five-minute break from working at your desk. When you sit down in a chair, try doing some chair squats before settling in. You can find ways to fit exercise into your life many times per day if a thirty-minute-plus chunk of time is just not something you can manage.

Adults who wish to lose weight and keep it off are likely to have to do an hour a day of exercise. The same applies here—you can divide this time into manageable short chunks.

MORE WORKOUTS FOR THE WHOLE FAMILY

Here, I'd like to supply you with four more resistance-training workouts that moms and dads (and kids!) can do pretty much anywhere. Along with the playground workout, these workouts can be mixed and matched to promote strength and fitness for everyone in your family, and with minimal equipment. They can be paired with either of the stretch series that have already appeared in these pages—the pregnancy/postpartum stretches on pages 50–54, or the playground stretches on pages 102–103. The freestyle and band exercises in the pregnancy/postpartum workout are also fair game here.

Each workout will take from fifteen to twenty minutes. Each will raise your heart rate enough to qualify as cardio work as well as strength training.

The first workout is a freestyle workout requiring no equipment at all.

The second uses a rubber resistance band—the same long, stretchy piece of tubing used in the pregnancy/postpartum workout on pages 44–49. (You may want to keep a few of these around in case your children want to join you in this workout.)

The third workout uses a stability ball, also known as a Swiss ball or balance ball, and a pair of light weights—three to five pounds should be plenty. These are available at any sporting goods store. The ball should be bought to match your height; its packaging should tell you how tall you should be to use that particular size.

And, finally, the last workout is a short advanced workout that really gets your heart rate up and builds a lot of strength in the legs. This one is especially good for hyperactive children who are stuck indoors on a rainy or snowy day!

FIFTEEN-MINUTE FREESTYLE HOME WORKOUT

Unless otherwise mentioned, do ten to fifteen reps of each exercise. You can do one set of each to begin with, and you can then add a second set as you become more fit. Perform each exercise slowly, so that momentum doesn't take over.

FREESTYLE DEADLIFT

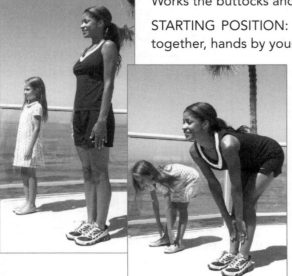

Works the buttocks and hamstrings.

STARTING POSITION: Stand tall with your feet together, hands by your sides.

ACTION: Looking out in front of you, begin to slide your hands down the front of your legs as you slightly bend your knees. Slide the hands to mid-shin level or to the tops of the feet. Reverse the movement to return to the starting position.

SINGLE-LEG DEADLIFT

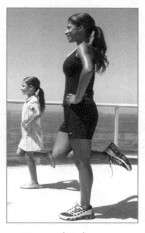

Works the buttocks and hamstrings.

STARTING POSITION: Stand on one foot, hands on hips. Lift the other leg, bending the knee so that the lower part of the lifted leg is parallel to the ground.

ACTION: Tilt your whole upper body forward, reaching both hands for the ground. At the same time, press the lifted leg up and back as though you were trying to put the sole of that foot on the ceiling. Then, reverse the movement to return to the starting position.

Keep looking out in front of you throughout the exercise; if balance is an issue, it may help to figure out a stationary spot to keep your eyes on throughout. Only use a wall or chair for support if you absolutely have to, and if you do, don't lean on it—just rest your hand or a finger or two there, gently. (The balancing component of

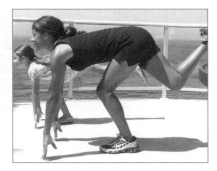

this exercise adds to its strengthening effects.) Do this exercise 10 times on one leg before switching feet and repeating 10 times on the other leg.

FREESTYLE SQUATS

Great conditioning for the whole lower body.

STARTING POSITION: Stand with hands on hips, feet shoulder-width apart. (See next page.)

ACTION: Squat your hips down and back, reaching both arms out in front of you. Keep your knees aligned with the direction in which your toes are pointing, and keep your heels on the floor. Think of trying to sit on a chair that's about four feet behind you! To finish, straighten the knees, stand up tall, and put hands back on the hips.

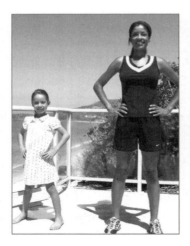 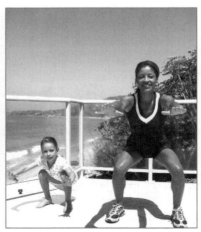

PUSH-UPS

Nothing beats them for upper body and core strengthening!

STARTING POSITION: You can begin in a standard push-up position with your hands and balls of the feet on the ground or on your hands with your knees on the ground. Either way, hold your body in a strong position, feeling the abs work. Shoulders are spread and tail is tucked. Hands are planted at least shoulder-width apart.

ACTION: Lower your chest toward the ground, stopping when the elbows reach a 90-degree angle. Reverse, straightening the elbows. Go to failure—that means, do as many as you can do with proper form!

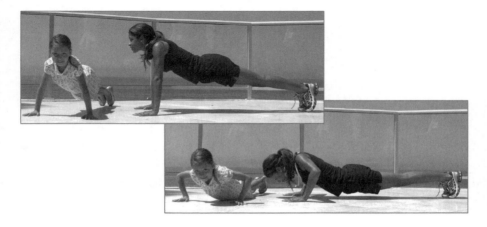

PILLAR BRIDGE

A great core strengthener.

STARTING POSITION/ACTION: Here, starting position and action are one and the same. Lie on your belly and put your forearms on the floor. Clasp

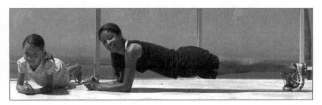

your hands and press your hips up so that you are in a plank position, resting only on the forearms and the balls of the feet.

Beginners, hold for 30 seconds; more advanced, hold 60 to 90 seconds.

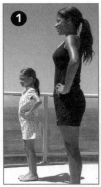

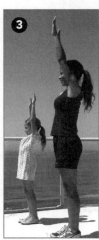

FRONT LUNGE WITH REACH AND PRESS

More lower-body strengthening with an added strength/endurance component for the arms and shoulders.

STARTING POSITION: Stand with feet together, hands on hips.

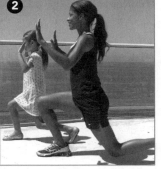

ACTION: This exercise happens in two parts.

First: Lunge out onto one leg, making sure that the heel of the lunging leg stays on the ground. Ideally, it should get to about a 90-degree angle at the knee. Drop the back knee toward the floor and reach the palms straight out in front of you as you lunge forward.

Second: As you return to the starting position, press both arms straight overhead. Return the hands to the hips before next repetition.

Do 10 repetitions each leg—you can alternate or do one leg at a time.

BURPEE

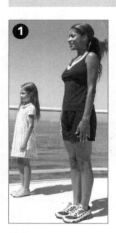

An allover conditioner and cardiovascular strengthener.

STARTING POSITION: Stand with feet together.

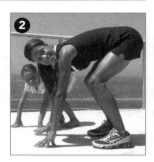

ACTION: Spread feet hip-width apart, then squat down and touch the ground with both hands. Jump back to a push-up position. Jump forward again into the squat. Then, stand up, reaching high with both arms. This is a tough one! Build up from 2 to 3 reps to 10 reps.

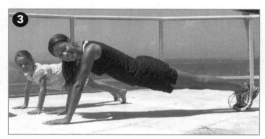

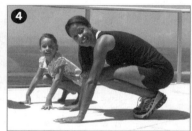

V-UP CRUNCH

An intense abdominal strengthener.

STARTING POSITION: Lie on your back with arms overhead and legs extended. (If you need to build basic strength, start out doing this exercise with knees bent and feet flat on the floor.)

ACTION: Take a big in-breath, and on the exhale, press both feet up to the ceiling as you reach for your toes. At the same time, lift your head and the tops of your shoulders off the floor. On the inhale, return to the starting position. If your abs aren't strong enough to do this yet, as suggested try starting with your knees bent and feet flat on the floor. Instead of lifting the feet to the ceiling, lift the knees. Do 15 to 25 reps.

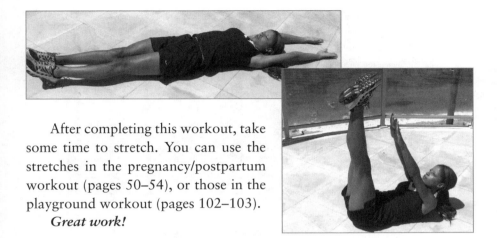

After completing this workout, take some time to stretch. You can use the stretches in the pregnancy/postpartum workout (pages 50–54), or those in the playground workout (pages 102–103).

Great work!

FIFTEEN- TO TWENTY-MINUTE RESISTANCE-BAND WORKOUT

This is a quick full-body resistance workout that can be done just about anywhere—in your office, living room, child's playroom, or even in your hotel room while traveling. To increase the resistance as you build strength, pull the resistance band tauter by winding it up in your hands. You may eventually want to invest in a few bands of different colors (indicating different levels of resistance) to give yourself an additional challenge.

ONE-ARM ALTERNATING BAND PRESS

Works the chest and triceps.

STARTING POSITION: Loop the band around something sturdy that is about chest height. Face away so that you will be pushing the band against resistance. Hold one handle in each hand at shoulder height, with the band extending over the tops of the shoulders. Gently squat, bending the knees slightly and leaning forward as though you were about to start running. (See next page.)

ACTION: Press one arm out in front of you, straightening the elbow completely. Let that arm bend back to the starting position as you extend the other arm. Do 15 repetitions per arm, alternating, for a total of 30 presses.

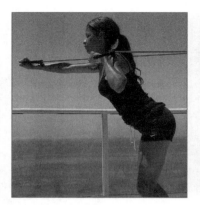
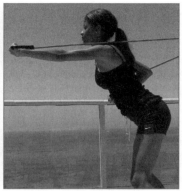

SQUAT AND BAND SHOULDER PRESS

For the lower body, shoulders, and arms.

STARTING POSITION: Stand with the band looped underneath both feet, holding one handle in each hand. Move your hands up so that they are at shoulder level and elbows are pointing down to the ground.

ACTION: This exercise happens in two parts.

First: Squat the hips down and back, keeping both heels on the floor. Try to reach a 90-degree angle at the knee joint. Return to the starting position.

Second: Press both hands straight overhead until the elbows are fully straight, then return the hands to the starting position. Repeat 10 to 15 times.

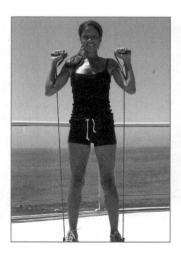
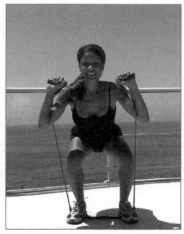

SQUAT + BAND ROWS

For the lower body, biceps, and upper back.

STARTING POSITION: Loop the band around something sturdy, like a post, a pillar, or the leg of a heavy table. Hold one handle in each hand and back away until your arms are extended out in front of you and the band is taut.

ACTION: This exercise happens in two parts.

First, squat: With feet hip-width apart, squat down, exhaling, until your legs are at a 90-degree angle with both heels planted firmly on the floor. Keep looking out in front of you to keep the back flat and long. As you inhale, straighten your knees again.

Second, row: Then, exhaling again, pull the band's handles toward you, keeping your elbows tucked and shoulders down, until your elbows are behind you and you feel your upper back muscles working. Inhale, let the arms straighten, and on your next exhale, squat again. Repeat 10 to 15 times.

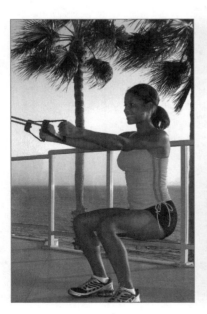
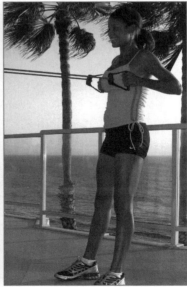

TRICEP AND BICEP BAND BLITZ

For the triceps, biceps, and lower body—this one hits them all.

STARTING POSITION: Loop the band around something low and sturdy. Step back until the band is taut.

ACTION: This exercise happens in two parts.

First, squat and tricep press: Squat your hips back, keeping your weight on your heels and your feet flat on the floor. Lean your torso way forward, keeping your arms at your sides. Straighten both arms, pressing them back until your hands are next to your hips and your elbows are straight.

Second, stand tall and bicep curl: In a smooth motion, without pausing, come out of your squat and stand up tall, leaning back slightly as you flip your hands so that palms face your front. Curl your hands up toward your shoulders, keeping elbows next to ribs. Repeat both steps for a total of 15 repetitions.

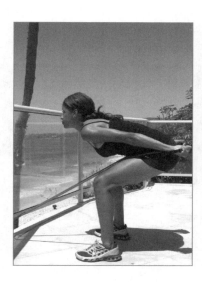 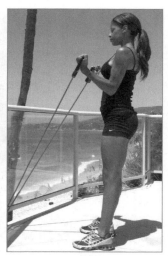

LATERAL PILLAR BRIDGE WITH ONE-ARM BAND ROW

For the core muscles (abdominals and back) and the latissimus dorsi (muscles that attach the arms to the spine).

STARTING POSITION: Loop the band around something sturdy and low. Sit down on the floor, facing the place you've looped the band, and far enough away that the band is taut. Stretch your body out on one side, resting the bottom elbow on the floor, then lift your hips up so that you are supporting all your weight on the bottom elbow and forearm and the outside edge of the bottom foot. The top arm should be extended out in front of you, holding the band's handle (or both handles).

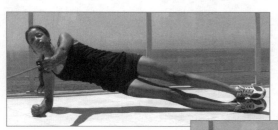

ACTION: Pull your elbow in so that it brushes your ribs. Draw that elbow as far back behind you as you can. Return to starting position.

Try for 10 to 12 reps on one side, holding the body straight and maintaining the 'bridge' throughout all 10 to 12 repetitions.

STATIONARY LUNGE WITH SINGLE-ARM ROW

For the lower and upper body.

STARTING POSITION: Loop the band around something sturdy that is about waist-high. Hold the band in your right hand and step back until the band is taut and your right arm is extended straight out in front of you. Place your left leg in front and right leg behind, setting up for your lunge.

ACTION: Drop your right knee straight down toward the ground as you bend your left knee to 90 degrees. At the same time, row back with your right arm so that the elbow comes right along the side of the ribs and presses back behind you; punch your left arm out in front of you as you row your right arm back. Return to starting position and repeat 10 to 15 times before switching legs.

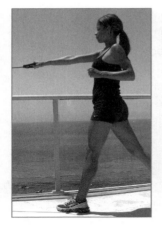
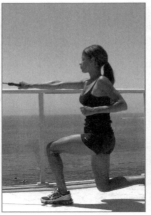
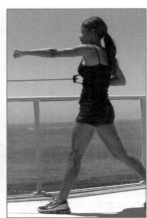

BICYCLE ABS

Targets the abdominal and oblique muscles (muscles that wrap around the sides of the waist).

STARTING POSITION: Lie face-up on the floor and lace your fingers behind your head. Bring your knees in toward your chest and lift your shoulder blades off the ground—without pulling on your head.

ACTION: Straighten the left leg out to about a 45-degree angle while simultaneously turning your upper body to the right. Bring left elbow toward right knee. Then, reverse, bringing left knee in and right elbow across toward the left knee. Repeat 10 to 15 times on both sides.

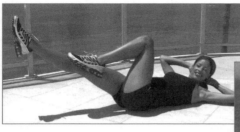

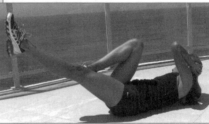

. . . and stretch! *Excellent work!*

FIFTEEN- TO TWENTY-MINUTE STABILITY BALL/DUMBBELL WORKOUT

Using a Swiss ball or a balance ball with a weight workout engages muscles throughout the body to stabilize the weight as you move it. This is a very efficient way to train the entire body, particularly the core muscles of the trunk.

DUMBBELL PRESS ON BALL

For the chest and triceps.

STARTING POSITION: Holding the weights, sit on the Swiss ball. Walk your feet out until your upper back and head are resting on the ball, both feet flat on the floor. Hold your weights as though you had a barbell in your hands, elbows out to the side.

ACTION: Press the dumbbells straight up, extending your elbows, until they meet over the center of your chest. Return to starting position. Repeat 15 to 20 times.

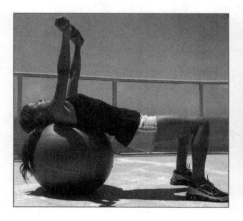 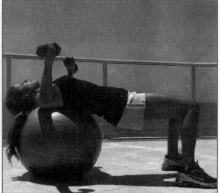

SWISS BALL ONE-ARMED DUMBBELL ROW

For the upper back, lats, and core.

STARTING POSITION: Stand with a dumbbell in your right hand and the Swiss ball slightly in front of you and off to the left. Leaning forward, place your left hand on the Swiss ball and let your right hand hang down. Walk your right foot 3 feet to the right of the ball, then lift your left foot about 12 inches off the floor and rest the knee on the ball. The Swiss ball will be slightly to the left of you when you work the right arm, and vice versa.

ACTION: Pull your right elbow up behind you in a rowing motion, passing the elbow next to your body. Lift the elbow as high as it will go, then return to starting position. Repeat 15 times before switching sides.

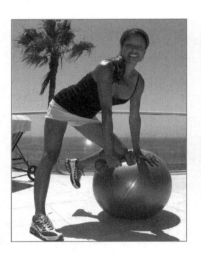 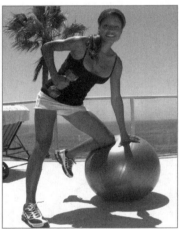

HAMSTRING LYING BALL FLEX

For the backs of the legs and buttocks.

STARTING POSITION: Lie down on your back with the ball under your lower legs. Press your hips up, making a bridge with your body from the floor to the ball. Keep your arms and hands on the floor.

ACTION: Keeping your hips lifted, bend the knees so that the ball rolls toward you. Keep bending the knees until the backs of your heels are resting on the top of the ball. Return to starting position.

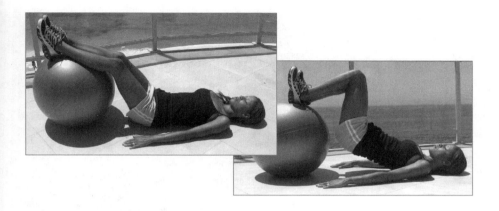

LYING BALL GLUTE BRIDGE

For the glutes!

STARTING POSITION: Lie on your back with your legs resting on the ball, feet together, arms at sides facing down.

ACTION: Lift your hips toward the ceiling. You will

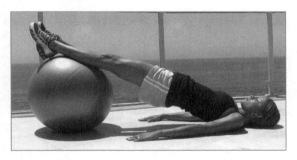

end up resting on your shoulders and arms with the back of your head on the floor. Stay there for 1 to 3 seconds, then lower the hips to the floor, returning to the starting position.

SWISS BALL SIT-UPS

For the abdominals.

STARTING POSITION: Lie on your back, placing your legs around the Swiss ball. Place your hands behind the top part of your neck. Keep your neck long, chin away from your chest, and elbows out to the sides. (See next page.)

ACTION: As you contract your abdominals to lift shoulders and head off the floor, lift the Swiss ball off the ground with your legs, pressing it toward your head. Repeat 15 to 25 times.

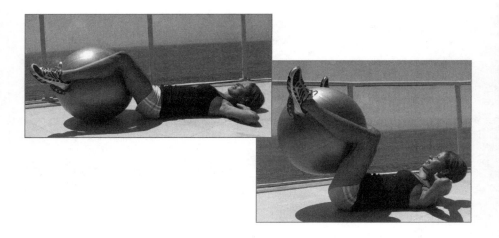

SWISS BALL OPPOSITES

Conditions the back muscles.

STARTING POSITION: Lie on your belly on top of the ball. Extend your arms and legs so that the tips of your toes and fingers are touching the ground.

ACTION: Exhale, lifting the left arm and the right leg toward the ceiling, gently—without jerking! Inhale, lower the left arm and the right leg; then repeat with the right arm and the left leg. Repeat 10 to 15 times on both sides.

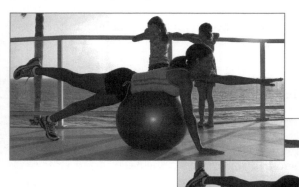

BALL SQUATS WITH DUMBBELL SHOULDER PRESS

Serious upper and lower body strengthening!

STARTING POSITION: Stand with the Swiss ball between you and a wall, a column, or some other immoveable object, at about waist height. Walk your feet out in front of you so that you are leaning your weight against the ball. Feet are shoulder-width apart. Hold the dumbbells in your hands at shoulder height.

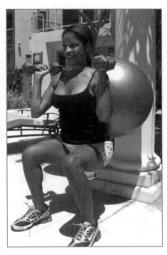

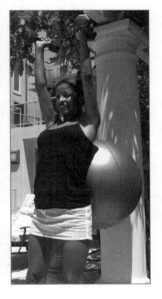

ACTION: This exercise happens in two parts.

First: Squat your hips straight down toward the floor, keeping your back straight as you roll it down the ball. Keep the dumbbells close to your shoulders.

Second: Return to starting position, straightening your knees. Press the dumbbells straight overhead; then, lower them back to the starting position. Repeat 15 times.

. . . take some time to stretch when you're done. *Great job!*

FIFTEEN-MINUTE ADVANCED WORKOUT

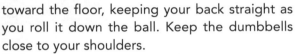

This is a workout to do once you've done the others regularly, plus cardio, at least four times weekly, for at least a couple of weeks. This is a good option when you are crunched for time or need to blow off some steam. You can also do this workout at the track or park after a walk. This workout exercises many of the major muscle groups all at once.

JUMP SQUATS

Begin with the legs in a wide stance (at least shoulder-width apart) in a squat, with your arms outstretched in front of you. Jump explosively, straight up, while reaching both arms overhead. Return to starting position. Work up to 15 repetitions.

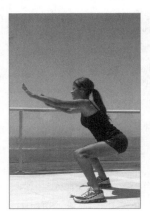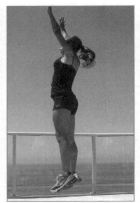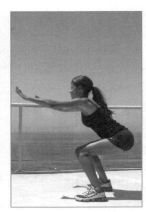

LATERAL (SIDE-TO-SIDE) JUMPS

Place two dumbbells on the ground, a few feet apart. Place them on their ends so that they're standing up. Squat down behind one of them and touch its end with your fingertips. Then, staying low in your squat, jump both legs to the side at once so that you are behind the other dumbbell. Touch it with your fingertips, then jump back to the first dumbbell. Work up to 10 repetitions.

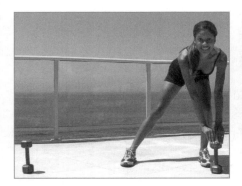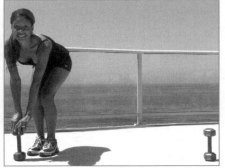

PUSH-UP BURPEE WITH JUMP

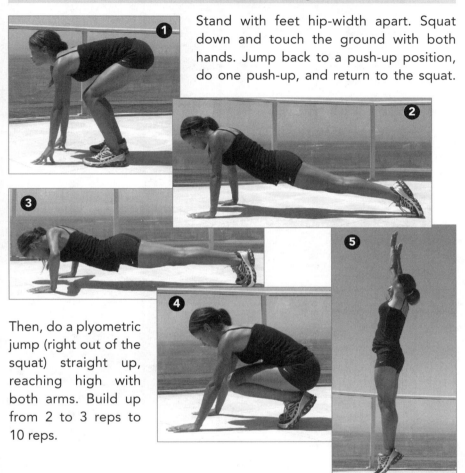

Stand with feet hip-width apart. Squat down and touch the ground with both hands. Jump back to a push-up position, do one push-up, and return to the squat.

Then, do a plyometric jump (right out of the squat) straight up, reaching high with both arms. Build up from 2 to 3 reps to 10 reps.

PLYOMETRIC JUMP LUNGES

Stand with feet hip-width apart. Then, step one leg a couple of feet in front of the other. (See next page.) From this position drop into a lunge, by dropping the back knee toward the floor and bending the front knee. Jump and switch the feet, putting the other foot forward and the other foot back, and lunge on that side. Let your arms move however they naturally want to move. Repeat 10 times. Keep your torso vertical throughout.

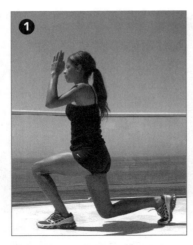
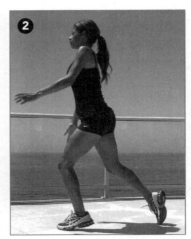
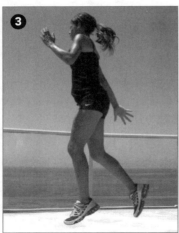
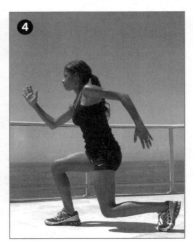

CROSSOVER V-UPS

Lie on your back on the floor, one leg straight and the other bent. Lift your head and shoulders off the floor. Tuck the same-side arm as the out-stretched leg behind your head and extend the opposite arm overhead. Lift your straightened leg up toward the ceiling; at the same time, reach for the lifted foot with your opposite hand. Return to starting position and repeat, lifting the same leg and reaching with the opposite arm. Repeat 15 times each side for a total of 30.

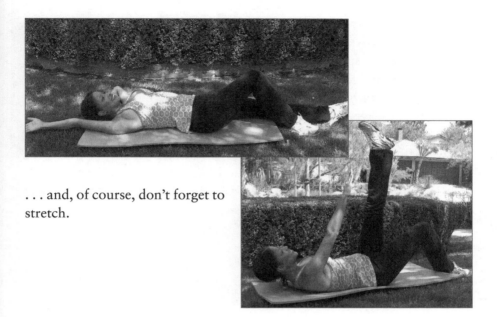

. . . and, of course, don't forget to stretch.

TO RECAP

Aim to do one of the four workouts (the playground workout or one of the three home workouts) at least three times per week. Do some kind of cardio on as many days a week as you can, especially on days when you don't do another workout. Enjoy the yoga exercises with your children or modify them to do on your own. Your child, as soon as she's able to follow along, probably will do so, no matter what workout you're doing—a great start for her lifetime of fitness.

FIT FAMILY WORKOUT TEACHABLE MOMENTS

If the child joins you for the strengthening part of any of these workouts, explain that working the muscles until they are tired will make them stronger, and may even make them bigger. Tell the child that making his arms stronger will help him to throw a ball farther and climb faster. That strengthening her legs will enable her to jump higher, execute her dance moves better, or play better soccer. Let the child see how these strengthening exercises will improve her skills at the things she really enjoys doing.

Let her know that making her heart beat fast, her lungs breathe deeper, and her body become warm or sweaty is helping to bring oxygen and nutrients to every single square inch of her body, inside and out, and that a strong heart and strong lungs will help her feel great all day long.

Use your creativity to find lots more teachable moments throughout your workouts, whether your children participate or not. The more they know, the more likely they'll be to join in.

After finishing an exercise session, ask the child how she feels. Ask her, "Do you have lots of energy? That's your body making special chemicals called *endorphins* that make you feel great and have extra energy after you exercise."

CHAPTER 6

Fit Family, Smart Family, Happy Family

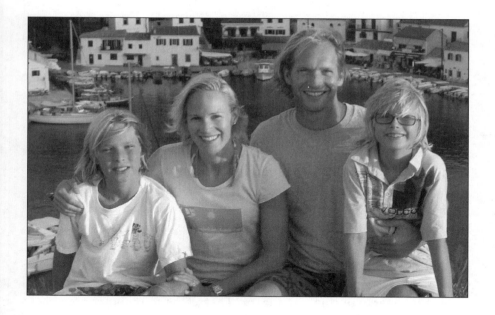

Most parents believe that academic achievement is important for success in life. Learning social skills and developing healthy relationships with family and friends are also held up as important aspects of well-being and all-around health and happiness. What's less obvious is the link between fitness and good nutrition and these aspects of well-being.

In recent years, research has begun to emerge that suggests that fitness and nutrition are closely linked to a child's social well-being and academic achievement. Researchers at the University of Illinois gave 259 third and fifth graders the standard physical fitness test: sit-and-reach, running, and sit-ups and push-ups against the clock. Once the results were tabulated, the researchers checked the children's physical fitness test scores against their standardized math and reading test scores. The more fit the child, the better their academic scores were.

In other studies, scientists found that they could bring about the growth of new brain cells—something once believed to be impossible—simply by putting people on a regular three-month regimen of cardio exercise. High-intensity exercise was found to increase the connections between brain cells (nerve cells that are also known as neurons), which—as writer Mary Carmichael wrote in *Newsweek* magazine—"form[s] dense, interconnected webs that make the brain run faster and more efficiently" ("Stronger, Faster, Smarter," March 26, 2007). So much for the stereotype of the dumb jock!

Schools that offer intense physical education programs see positive effects on academic achievement, students' ability to concentrate, test scores in writing, reading, and math, and reduced disruptive behavior—even when P.E. offerings cut into time offered for academics (Tufts University Center on Hunger, Poverty and Nutrition Policy, Statement on the Link Between Nutrition and Cognitive Development in Children, Medford, MA: 1994). Unfortunately, most public schools are cutting down on intense P.E. programs and putting kids in chairs in classrooms more often instead of the reverse. It falls to families to make up for lost physical activity time.

Nutrition is as important as exercise for children's academic achievement and brain development. A child whose nutritional needs are met will have more energy to think and learn. They come to school more able to absorb information. Good nutrition also means better immune system function, which translates to less time spent out sick, missing important classwork.

Many studies have demonstrated a connection between poor nutrition and disciplinary and behavioral problems. A good breakfast that includes protein (from dairy, nut butters, eggs, or meat) is especially helpful for children's focus at school.

Here's a big Fit Family suggestion for great academic and interpersonal achievement: family dinners. When families collaborate in creating menus, shopping, preparing meals, and sitting down together (facing each other, not facing a TV) over dinner for good conversation, *teachable moments* are everywhere! Family dinners at least five times weekly positively affect a child's academic achievement, lower risk of alcohol, drug, or tobacco use, and more. You'll find a complete section on family dinners later in this chapter.

From the earliest beginnings of life, children moving their bodies in developmentally appropriate ways will impact the child's intelligence and emotional and social development. Let's explore how this happens even in infancy.

THE 'CONTINUUM CONCEPT' AND OPTIMAL CHILD DEVELOPMENT

A sociologist named Jean Liedloff spent several years studying a South American tribe called the *Yequana*. They were very primitive, still living as though they were in the Stone Age. Ms. Liedloff's primary interest ended up being how amazingly calm, obedient, and self-reliant their children were, and how quickly they were able to take on responsibilities within the tribe. Infants in this tribe almost never cried. What were the Yequana doing that we weren't in the United States?

The result of her research was a book called *The Continuum Concept* (Da Capo Press, rev. ed. 1986), which outlines how infants in this tribe were always in the arms of or lying next to an adult (usually, the mother) or other caregiver until they were able to scoot around on their own— usually, around seven or eight months of age. There's more to this concept than just being held, and the book is worth looking at if you are about to become a mother. In an article for *Mothering* magazine, published in winter 1989, Ms. Liedloff realized something else about this "in-arms" phase:

> One can very quickly calm a fussing baby by running or jumping with the child, or by dancing or doing whatever eliminates one's own energy excess. A mother or father who must suddenly go out to get

something need not say, "Here, you hold the baby. I'm going to run down to the shop." The one doing the running can take the baby along for the ride. The more action, the better!

. . . A baby seething with undischarged energy is asking for action: a leaping gallop around the living room or a swing from the child's hands or feet. The baby's energy field will immediately take advantage of an adult's discharging one. Babies are not the fragile things we have been handling with kid gloves. In fact, a baby treated as fragile at this formative stage can be persuaded that he or she is fragile.

By taking your baby with you *on your body,* not in a stroller, you are giving that baby invaluable stimulation for the development of his nervous system. You are soothing him, too, and filling his need for body-to-body human contact. He hears your heartbeat, feels your warmth and the subtle (and not-so-subtle) movements of your body, and hears and feels the vibration of your voice. There is no righter place for an infant to be than snuggled up against the body of a caregiver.

In the earliest months of life, an infant receives most of his nervous system stimulation through touch. That stimulation is key for proper physical, mental, and emotional development. Being touched and carried strongly affects the baby's *vestibular system.* The vestibular system is the part of the nervous system that coordinates and modifies information that comes in through the senses of hearing, seeing, and the child's sense of his or her own body in space. Vestibular stimulation is instrumental for developing physical coordination and balance, and a baby who is held most of the time he or she is awake is getting constant vestibular stimulation.

One great way to soothe a fussy baby, as most parents know, is through rocking, jostling, and bouncing. Some mothers find that the only thing that will calm a colicky baby is to sit on a Swiss ball, hold him tight, and bounce up and down as hard as she can! Bouncing, rocking, and jostling are soothing for most babies, and this is because infants naturally crave vestibular stimulation. Many older children also enjoy being wrestled with, tickled, bounced, and hugged roughly, because this continues that process of nervous system development.

When parents or other caregivers hold and carry the infants in their charge throughout most of the first eight or nine months of life, they are fostering secure attachment between child and adult. Secure attachment to caregivers, which is established in the first year of life through being picked up, held, and fed on demand (not only by the mother or father, but also by any caregiver), promotes better emotional, social, and cognitive health later on. According to developmental psychologist Aletha Solter, Ph.D., author of several books, including *The Aware Baby* (Shining Star Press, rev. ed. 2001) and *Raising Drug-Free Kids* (Da Capo Press, 2006), children who are securely attached at one year of age tend to be more confident, independent, socially competent, curious, and empathic when age four or five.

If you use proper ergonomics and a good carrier, your back, shoulders, and neck will be up to the task. And you'll have the enjoyment of feeling your baby up against you, being in constant touch with his needs. With many carriers, mom can even nurse discreetly while on the move. You can wear your baby around the house while doing chores or going to the grocery store, too, and have both hands free—far easier than a stroller.

To choose the right carrier for you and for your baby, go to a baby supply store or do a Web search for "baby carrier" or "baby sling," or check out the following websites: http://sutemigear.com or www.theslingstation.com. Choose a carrier that holds the baby against your body, and that can be used in different positions. Moms I know have recommended the Maya Wrap sling, which comes in attractive colors and patterns, and the Over the Shoulder Baby Holder sling, which has more padding.

Slings are a good choice because they can be worn on either shoulder and can be used for every age of your baby, from newborn (lying down) to the toddler years (holding the toddler against your hip, so you have your hands free). Dr. Solter and others claim that when a baby is held straddling the caregiver's hip, it promotes proper hip joint development and gives appropriate stimulation to the child's developing nervous system. A sling can also be loosened and slipped off over mom's head to put a sleeping baby down on a bed or crib, right inside the sling. I've also been told that the sling may be hard to get the hang of at first, but those who keep at it end up very happy with it.

Some moms I've talked to also like the Ergo baby carrier, which is a soft carrier that can be worn on the front or back and can hold baby facing out or in.

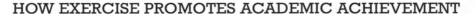

HOW EXERCISE PROMOTES ACADEMIC ACHIEVEMENT

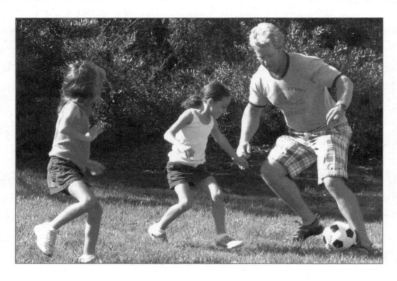

So, let's say your child has gotten through this in-arms phase and well into his preschool or elementary school years. How does adhering to the family workouts in Chapter 5 and otherwise trying to ensure that the child gets an hour of exercise most days of the week promote better achievement for that child in school?

Here's what the scientists say about this:

- When your child gets aerobic exercise, the heart pumps more blood to the muscles—and to the brain. A good cardio workout means better brain cell oxygenation.

- Nutrients (including carbohydrates, fats, protein, vitamins, and minerals) are carried in the bloodstream. More blood pumping through the brain also means more nutrients pumping through.

- There is a direct connection between the repetitive muscle contractions of exercise and the ability of the brain to absorb new information. Every time a muscle contracts, it sends out chemicals that directly affect the brain's production of neurotransmitters and *growth factors*. One growth factor, *brain-derived neurotrophic factor* (BDNF), has been called "Miracle-Gro for the brain" by Harvard psychiatrist John Ratey. It stimulates the branching out of nerve cells, which leads to better communication

Do Mom's or Dad's Brains Sprout New Connections and Neurons with Exercise?

Definitely, yes. Even though adults tend to lose neurons as they age, you can stimulate your body to generate new neurons in brain areas important for learning, memory, decision-making, multi-tasking, and thinking ahead by exercising (both physically and mentally). However, these effects of exercise on the brain are more pronounced in children than in grownups.

- Athletes have higher activity of specialized brain cells called *astrocytes*, which mop up "used" neurotransmitters, thereby helping neurons to function better.

- Dopamine, serotonin, and norepinephrine—neurotransmitters that sustain balanced mood, focus, and attention span—are all elevated after a bout of exercise. Frequent exercise maintains this balance over time. John Ratey, M.D., says that a bout of exercise is "like taking a little bit of Prozac and a little bit of Ritalin" because it calms, focuses, lifts mood, and tones down impulsivity.

- Cultivating an early love of physical activity may protect your child, in much, much later years, against the cognitive downhill slide that is too often seen in today's aging people: first with mild cognitive impairment, then Alzheimer's disease. People who exercise more often are stimulating their brains in ways that reduce their risk of these conditions.

- Depression is a growing problem in American youth, with an estimated 10 to 15 percent of the child and adolescent population in the United States suffering from some form of depressive disorder at any given time. And exercise, as it turns out, is an antidepressant on par with the medications often prescribed to treat depressive disorders. Some experts even think that depression might be a symptom of a body—and, by association, a brain—that isn't being used for the purposes for which it was designed: not to sit in front of screens, in cars, and in chairs all day, but to be active!

between those cells—the same thing that happens when we learn new information and "hardwire" it into the brain. Higher BDNF levels mean greater capacity for learning.

FOOD, ACHIEVEMENT, AND BEHAVIOR

In the United States, we are fortunate enough to have enough food to keep just about every child adequately fed. But children who turn their noses up at whole, natural foods can easily end up malnourished—not enough to make them sick or show outright signs of deficiency, but enough to affect their performance in school and their behavior at school and at home. Multiple studies show that even slight, *subclinical* deficiency of essential vitamins and minerals or of dietary protein has an impact on academic performance, behavior, and intelligence in children. And even a child who is overweight or obese from a calorie-rich, nutrient-poor diet can have this outcome.

Studies have shown that adding a daily multivitamin/mineral supplement to the diet of a child who has not been well nourished brings improvements in academic performance and behavior, and may also help boost energy for physical activity. Check with your child's pediatrician about which type of "multi" he or she thinks is best. *More is not better* when it comes to vitamin supplements, so do *not* give a child an adult supplement! (Keep all supplements out of reach of children. Iron overdose from nutritional supplements is one of the most common causes of poisoning in children under the age of five.)

Certain nutrients are more likely to be lacking and affecting the child's behavior or school performance.

Iron

Iron deficiency is a common issue, affecting about 9 percent of toddlers, ages one to two, and about 9 to 11 percent of adolescent girls and women. Breastfed infants are at higher risk of iron deficiency than formula-fed infants, because the amount of iron that goes into the mother's milk depends on her own stores of this nutrient. Iron deficiency in children is most common during periods of rapid growth.

If your child has symptoms of iron deficiency (pale skin, lips, hands, or eyelids; irritability; lack of energy or fatigues easily; high heart rate; sore or swollen tongue; or an urge to eat dirt or other things that aren't food), you may want to check in with your pediatrician for a blood test.

Foods rich in iron include meat, poultry, fish, leafy greens such as kale and cabbage, beans, and whole grains. Iron supplements for children are available, but don't give one of these to your child unless your doctor recommends it.

Protein

One study of fourth graders found that kids with the lowest protein intake had the lowest academic achievement scores. The average child's breakfast is very high in carbs but lacking in protein, which balances blood sugar and gives sustained energy throughout the morning. School breakfast programs often offer a source of protein, and this is why kids who struggle academically and then go on these programs usually begin to do better.

Try to include a good concentrated source of protein in your child's breakfast—for that matter, in every meal. A big, hearty breakfast is a great start to your child's day. Try the following:

- Scrambled eggs or nut butter on a whole-wheat English muffin or bagel.

- A protein smoothie made with plain yogurt, protein powder, juice, and frozen fruit.

- A turkey burger with a small amount of cheese melted on top, cut up on a plate with fresh fruit on the side.

Shake up your preconceptions about breakfast! You don't have to feed your child cereal with milk or a bagel with cream cheese—you can even try soup, leftovers from last night's dinner, or cubed cheese, whole-grain crackers, and sliced fruit. (For more ideas, see the recipes at the end of the book.)

Calcium/Magnesium/Vitamin D

A study presented at the American Academy of Pediatrics' 2003 meeting revealed a shockingly high incidence of osteoporosis *in children, ages six to thirteen.* That's right—although most of us think of osteoporosis as a disease of elderly women, it can begin in childhood. The study followed 447 children, ages six to thirteen, who had broken a bone in what should have been a minor fall or other injury-causing event. Of these children, a subset had had more than one break, and they were given a bone density scan. *Sixty-seven percent* of these children had osteoporosis.

Childhood is prime bone-building time. The more bone your child builds during these years, the lower his or her risk of osteoporosis throughout her lifetime. Calcium, vitamin D, magnesium, and protein are all nutritional ingredients needed to build bone. (Regular physical activity is just as important.) Statistics show that many children do not meet the daily requirements for calcium, magnesium, or vitamin D intake.

Daily childhood calcium requirements are as follows:

- Ages one to three: 500 milligrams (mg)

- Ages four to eight: 800 mg

- Ages nine to thirteen: 1,300 mg

- Ages fourteen to eighteen: 1,300 mg

Good food sources of calcium include yogurt, vitamin D-fortified milk and orange juice, cheese, leafy greens, legumes, and nuts.

Daily childhood magnesium requirements:

- Infants six months to one year: 75 mg

- Ages one to three: 80 mg

- Ages four to eight: 130 mg

- Ages nine to thirteen: 240 mg

- Adolescent females, ages fourteen to eighteen: 360 mg

- Adolescent males, ages fourteen to eighteen: 410 mg

Good food sources of magnesium are green vegetables, whole grains, legumes, almonds, and fish.

Vitamin D is a nutrient found in food, but also is made in the skin when sunshine strikes it (without sunscreen in the way). Children growing up in northern latitudes are at risk of deficiency because of this lack of sunshine. So are those who have dark skin (African Americans, Hispanics, Asians), as their skin has more natural UV-blocking pigment.

For breastfed babies who do not get daily sunshine on their skin, and for children or adolescents who don't get ten minutes of direct sun most days or who don't drink at least 17 ounces of vitamin D-fortified milk per day, a supplement containing 200 IU (international units) per day is advised by most pediatricians.

Good food sources of vitamin D include fish and eggs. White button mushrooms, when put out into UV light for a while, make a huge amount of vitamin D, and can be a good source of this nutrient for children who like them.

FAMILY DINNERS AND OTHER FIT FAMILY TRADITIONS

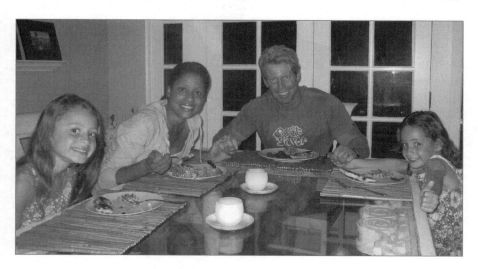

If there were a "magic bullet" that could help reduce your children's risk of obesity, drug/alcohol abuse, hospitalization, and emotional instability, would you want to take advantage of it?

Here's the good news—there is such a magic bullet. It's called the *family dinner.*

In the typically chaotic life of the two-working-parent household, dinner time is especially precious—maybe the only time all day when everyone can spend time together, deepening their bonds and sharing what's happened in their day. But it's in these households that the family dinner most often seems to fall by the wayside.

What happened? As parents both tend to spend more time working, the time and energy they have for a family meal is less than it could be. Preparing a healthy meal from scratch is hard work and takes a lot more time than many parents feel they have in a day. Once families get used to the more addictive tastes of fast food and restaurant food, a home-cooked meal can seem bland in comparison.

As children get older and become more involved in homework assignments, social engagements, extracurricular activities and sports, fast food and microwave meals and bowls of cereal replace what used to be a nightly ritual of sitting down together at home and eating a healthy, complete meal together.

Miriam Weinstein, author of a book called *The Surprising Power of Family Meals: How Eating Together Makes Us Smarter, Stronger, Healthier and Happier* (Steerforth, 2006), has an interesting perspective on this problem. She writes, "We are living in a time of intense individualism in a culture defined by competition and consumption. It has become an article of faith that a parent's job is to provide every child with every opportunity to find his particular talent, interest, or bliss." She goes on to point out that this quest to highlight each child's individualism is good, of course, but it can push the family's precious together time out of the picture—and that this is not something we can afford to lose.

At the family meal, children learn important skills. They learn how to communicate and converse; how to listen to others; and how to share the events, trials, and tribulations of the day. When children participate in meal planning, shopping, and preparation, you'll find a wealth of *teachable moments*. Plenty of those moments will come up during the family meals as well.

In all the fun you'll have cooking with your children, don't forget the most important ingredient of all: the whole family, sitting down together, talking and laughing—and, hopefully, helping with the dishes when it's all done!

Becoming a fitter family is all about creating this and other traditions.

So many of the traditions families once observed have fallen out of our chaotic lives, and this is one reason we have such issues with overweight and obesity. Here are some other ideas for healthful family traditions:

- Family breakfasts.

- An after-dinner, after-dishes family walk.

- A Sunday outing to the park for games and a healthy picnic.

- A family or neighborhood game of basketball, touch football, volleyball, or soccer once a week.

- Grow a garden together—this is a great way to instill appreciation for veggies, fruits, and herbs, and can be done even in the smallest apartment setting.

- Or join a neighborhood vegetable gardening group or Consumer Supported Agriculture (CSA) group, which involves contributing both money and work time on a farm for a share of the harvest—see the link to the American Community Gardening Association on page 66 to start your own community garden.

- A thirty-minute family dance party in the living room once a week.

- Family yoga stretches before breakfast (see pages 103–112 to review those stretches).

- Before-bed tickle fights! (Belly laughter is a great abdominal workout and really gets the breathing muscles working!)

- The playground workout or the other family workouts described in Chapter 5.

    . . . fill in your own traditions here!

CHAPTER 7

Secrets of Fit, Energized Families

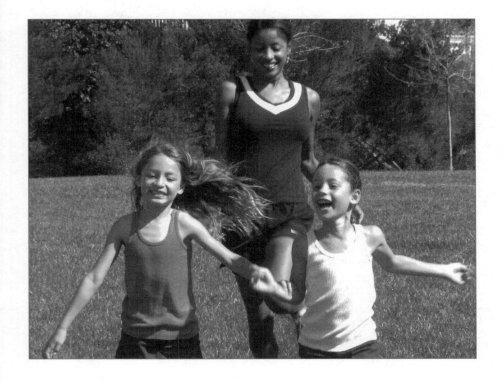

Sometimes, it just takes a small, simple tip from a parent who's already living a Fit Family Lifestyle to move others more in that direction. In this short chapter, I'll share with you some of these kinds of tips.

TIPS FOR STAYING FIT AND ENERGIZED

Some of the following ideas come from my own family habits; others were gathered from clients of mine who have figured out their own tips and tricks for staying fit and energized in the midst of the chaos of working, running their households, and raising their children.

Find Out Where Your Local Parks Are and Frequent Them

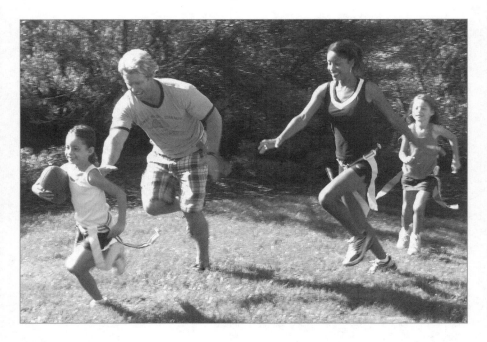

I'm always stunned to find that families who live in our area often don't know where the parks are. Find your own local parks. When the weather is agreeable, you and your children can spend lots of time there, playing, picnicking, and spending quality family time.

Our friend Douglas tells us that they make it a goal to do something physical every night after dinner, particularly in the summer. They might go to the park and take a ball, play chase, kick the ball around under the pretense that they're practicing soccer, climb ladders, slide down slides. "Anything—for at least thirty minutes. It is our bonding time. It gets everyone outdoors and active, and tires the kids out so that they sleep better."

Living in Southern California, sometimes we forget that in many parts of the United States, park play is strictly a summertime adventure. If you live in a place that gets a lot of cold, snowy weather, seek out community centers, YMCAs, or other places where kids and parents can get out of the house and get active as a family.

Create a Structured Regimen of Fitness Activities for Parents and Children

At our house, we have what I call the "Keeling Weekly Regimen." We find that scheduling everyone's fitness activities and putting them up on a week-long calendar doesn't feel so much like a limitation as it feels like our holding our physical fitness up as a priority.

Mom's workouts, dad's workouts, the kids' sports activities—they're all on there. Saturdays are our family active days; we go to the park, take walks, and play sports together. We often do some of this on Sundays, too, but we like to carve that out as a more restful day.

Try a "Shift Mentality" to Make Sure That Mom and Dad Get the Exercise They Need

Clarke, a pastor at Laguna Beach's Church By the Sea, has made fitness a priority for himself, and he makes sure his wife can do the same. "Staying physically fit is of high value in our family," he told me. "We appreciate both the physical benefits of being in shape and the mental energy and emotional outlet that training provides."

He and his wife have found, since having children, that getting to the gym regularly is much more of a challenge. "We have had to resort to some pretty tricky and flexible scheduling tactics to fit it all in. My wife and I utilize the 'shift' mentality when it comes to taking care of the babies. When it is my shift, she is free to work out or rest or do what she needs to do. Her free time then usually consists of a quick cardio workout, an abs routine, and then a sprint to the nearest latte stand and/or manicure and pedicure salon. When it is her turn to take the shift and mine to run free, I invariably head for the gym—unless there are waves, in which case I grab my board and head for the beach. The tricky thing is that my shift usually ends between three and four o'clock in the morning. How do I work out when I can hardly keep my eyes open? Frankly, I just gotta do it, and the character that is instilled as a result is worth every bit as much as the physical effects I gain from the training. So, the shift idea seems to work pretty well as long as you are flexible enough to squeeze that workout in between grocery runs and diaper changes. Either way, it's good for the mind, soul, and spirit."

Change the Way You Think and Talk about Food

Sure, food is an important aspect of culture and a major part of most celebrations. Some foods are so comforting—it's hard not to create a strong link between our favorite foods and feelings of pleasure and comfort.

Although there will always be holiday dinners and late-night brownie-baking memories that give us a nice warm feeling, we can be more conscious about the connections between eating and pleasure. When we do choose to eat because we want comfort or social time, we can still use moderation and be consciously aware of the real reward: precious time with people we love. And when our children are involved in occasions where food and celebration or comfort are being linked, take care to point out aspects of enjoyment aside from the food: "Isn't it great to spend time as a family?" instead of "Isn't it great to pig out on chocolate cake?" For some of these food-related family traditions, you can begin to substitute different activities (a walk or bike ride, or even a family touch football game) and new, healthier foods (for example, try some new recipes for Christmas or Thanksgiving dinner that are lower in fat and calories and high in healthful, nutrient-packed vegetables).

At the everyday level, however, we can shift our thinking from "eat to fill my belly" or "eat because I'm stressed" to "eat for fuel for my body" or "eat for fuel for great performance." We can talk this way to our children about food. "Okay, gang, it's time for breakfast—time to fuel up for a day of sharp thinking and plenty of running around!"

Cook as a Family—And Let Each Meal Be a Chance to Educate Your Children

Our friend Laura tells me that cooking as a family is an important part of helping their seven-year-old daughter, Sarah, to understand about portion size and the various food groups and their values. "We also have a rule that the kids have to try everything . . . it's really helped us to get the kids to try different types of food, even exotic foods like Thai food or sushi." Laura sees these exotic meals as an opportunity to learn about the cultures from which those foods come. "Fast food isn't part of any culture!" she told me.

Create a Home Environment Conducive to Family Fitness

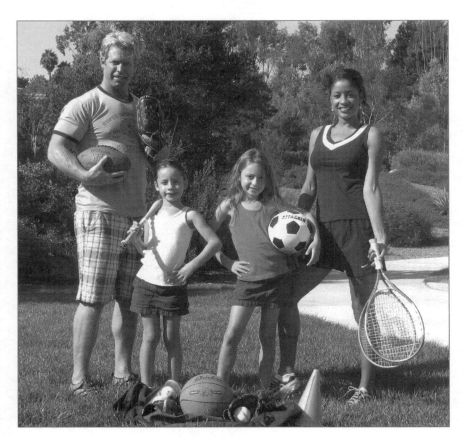

Over the years since the birth of our first child, Nikki and I have gathered a huge variety of sports equipment: tennis balls and rackets; Wiffle balls, Wiffle bats, a homemade plastic T-ball stand, and mitts; soccer balls; Hula-hoops; basketballs; Frisbees; badminton sets; jump ropes, and more. All the equipment was inexpensive and gathered over the years, some of it at yard sales—so there wasn't any big expenditure involved. We keep this equipment packed in a couple of duffle bags in the garage. When it's time to head out to the park or to the track, Nikki or I toss one of these bags into the car. We find that having equipment handy gets our girls more active and gives us more options for playing together actively as a family.

Nikki loves tennis, and on a Saturday, we often take the girls to the tennis courts to hit a few balls back and forth. When they get tired of it, they go to the playground right next to the tennis court to enjoy the play structure, and Nikki and I usually get at least a half-hour's worth of play in ourselves while keeping an eye on the girls. Sometimes the girls stop playing to watch the two of us!

Our friends Karla and Chris love to head to the track with their kids: "Sometimes we will go to the high school track, and run or walk or do the bleachers, and encourage the kids to do so. They don't always agree to running around the track, but they will play soccer or throw the baseball around, and hopefully see that physical activity is important for all of us . . . Other times we take them to different bike trails, either along the river or near the beach. They get to ride their bikes as we run. At the beach, we take walks and go for swims. This past year, Chris ran the L.A. Marathon. The kids and I watched him finish, and ever since then our youngest has been talking about running a marathon (in several years) . . . Having them see us exercising and enjoying it encourages them to do the same. We try and make fitness fun, and appeal to things they enjoy, and hope that they develop a lifelong enjoyment of physical activity."

Don't Skip Breakfast

When kids skip breakfast, they can end up tired, restless, and irritable. They won't function well without fueling up following their eight- to ten-hour overnight fast. Make breakfast a protein-rich meal whenever possible: include eggs, lean meats, yogurt, nut butter, or cheese.

As for you: skipping a meal almost always means you end up overeating at the next one. And did you know that sumo wrestlers have a little trick they use to put on extra pounds? That's right—they skip breakfast, to slow their metabolisms down a few extra notches. Enough said.

Try Cycling and Other Sports as a Family

The kids will love cycling with you. We started out with bike trailers that attached to our adult bikes, but now the girls are big enough to keep up on their own two-wheelers.

Our friend David tells me that his weekly workouts at the gym and his healthy eating habits give him the energy he needs to be an active participant in his son Merick's life. They walk around the block, swim at their local high school pool, and visit parks for outdoor play on the weekends. "My child will learn from me what it means to live an active, healthy lifestyle where exercise and proper nutrition are part of everyday life . . . it's important for me to maintain my health so that I may be an active participant in his future endeavors."

Try a New Approach to Discipline

Now, I'm completely against corporal punishment, but I've discovered one way to discipline our girls that is definitely physical. I was skeptical about it at first, but it works like a charm.

This idea came from another friend who is also named David. "Our household has incorporated physical activities into discipline," he told me. "The traditional time-out frequently requires too much time and certainly doesn't help with a child's extra energy. We have incorporated a program that when the children are not getting along they may be required to perform push-ups, sit-ups, or six-count burpees. When the kids have really been at each other, they run laps in the backyard with ten push-ups in between each lap. They usually find a way to get along afterwards. The kids are very good-natured about it, usually they end up laughing while they do it, and they much prefer that over a time-out."

Since my girls love to exercise, they're quick to redirect the energy that was going into fighting or rule-breaking and to put it whole-heartedly into doing their reps. By the time they're done, their mood has usually changed a great deal.

David does some other great things to help give his kids optimum nutrition. "I make fresh vegetable juice for the kids every day—about 8 ounces of kale, red chard, spinach, celery, zucchini, cucumber, and a very small amount of carrots or beets to reduce bitterness. They complain about it, but they also brag to their friends that their dad makes them drink fresh vegetable juice . . . The kids also get fresh fruit every day for snacks. At lunch and dinner, they start with fresh vegetables followed by protein (usually poultry or fish), followed by carbs (usually quinoa or rice, occasionally spelt pasta or whole-grain bread). Desserts are only served on the weekends. Sodas and juices are reserved for friends' birthday parties. Eliminating juices and desserts during the week has dramatically improved their dental checkups!" Not surprisingly, this fit dad keeps his kids active in sports, with swimming in the summer, basketball during the school year, three ski trips a year, and summer hikes in the mountains—average, five miles a day!

This unique disciplinary approach works really well with adults, too. Next time you're having a lousy day, and you're ready to lose your temper or make a choice you know isn't a good one, try giving yourself this kind of redirection. A few moments later, your heart rate's up, your face is flushed, and your mood is changed for the better.

Introduce Your Children to the Sports You Loved in Your Own Youth

Most of us played at least one sport or did some other physical activity as a child. Whether you played baseball (like I did), tennis, or basketball, swam competitively, twirled a baton, wrestled, did kung fu, or took ballroom dancing classes—it's never too early to introduce your favorite sport or activity to your children.

My friend Jeff told me about how he has managed this in his own busy life. He had been very athletic, engaging in running, lifting, and surfing from his early teens, but running his business had taken precedence over his workouts by his thirties. "Then, my wife, Jeri, signed us up with a family membership at the local gym and inspired me with the level of fitness that she had achieved by working out for an hour a day, Monday through Friday." By devoting six to eight hours per week to working out at the gym, Jeff was able to keep fit, but it wasn't until his son, Nile, became his workout partner that the workouts really became fun. "Nile has been a serious swimmer since he was ten, and was always intrigued by the machines in the gym. At thirteen, he started lifting light weights, with only a couple of exercises per session. Now, after two years of progressing, we spend two hours, five days a week exercising together. We have fun helping each other, and we have a friendly competition between us—he knows that I enjoy him being on the verge of overtaking me with his strength and endurance."

This father and son find that they have great personal and philosophical discussions—as well as moments for joking around—in rest periods during their workouts. "Often, these discussions are extended to others in the gym, which is in itself a close-knit community of interesting people. Nile is comfortable asking advice from trainers and other members about all kinds of subject matter." Jeff is grateful that Nile gets to hear so many wise and differing perspectives—and that his son is enjoying good health, extra energy, self-confidence, self-esteem, and a closer relationship with his dad as a result of these workouts.

Step Up the Drama at the Dinner Table

When I'm eating my vegetables in front of my girls, I make a *really big deal* over it. "Mmmmm," I say, rubbing my tummy and making my eyes big, "that broccoli tastes soooooo good, and I can feel how it's making my muscles stronger!" Now, even Kianna, my previously vegetable-averse younger daughter does the same thing. She eats her vegetables without any prodding and tells me eagerly that she can feel it in her muscles.

Kids love high drama, especially when it makes them laugh. Find ways to bring out your own dramatic flair during family meals to convey the value of "everyday foods" and you'll find your children naturally gravitating to those foods. After hearing enough times about how much stronger I felt after eating spinach (with the visual aid of me flexing my muscles), even Kianna was willing to give that green stuff a try!

Stay positive, and try to make your children laugh! Never try to bribe or force your children to eat their vegetables—or anything else, for that matter. It's their choice, no matter how you slice it. If they reject what you serve, remove it without any fuss, and don't offer a replacement. If you do, they'll start to treat you like a restaurant cook instead of a parent, expecting endless alternatives at mealtime if they don't like what everyone else is having. They'll come around.

Did I Mention That You Should Keep Refined Sugar Out of the House?

The road to obesity, diabetes, high blood pressure, heart disease, acne, mood disorders, attention deficit disorder, and even cancer is believed to be paved, in part, by sugar. Just get it out of your house—all the soft drinks, sweetened cereals, pastries, candy, and cookies.

When It's Gift Time, Try to Give Something That Encourages Physical Activity

When I was growing up, my grandpa used to come up with these kinds of gifts each Christmas. Instead of some toy that would have just sat in the corner, one year he gave us skis and lift tickets—which led to a new family tradition of heading up to the Sierras to go skiing. I've never forgotten his example, and now we try to come up with gift ideas for our girls that will help them get and stay active—sporting equipment or a trip to the water park, for example.

Fool the Eye with Small Plates

A sandwich on a dinner plate looks lost; on an appetizer plate, the same sandwich looks downright hefty.

Keep Looking for Ways to Make Family Meals Fun

Try having a picnic in the backyard when the weather is nice—or a picnic indoors on a blanket in the living room when the weather's not so nice!

We love to watch football as a family, so we'll sometimes have a football-themed meal and enjoy dinner in front of the game—the only time we watch TV during our family dinners. You might create a themed meal based on something your child loves: princesses, a certain movie, the season, or a cartoon character. Think of this as another place you can flex your creative muscles as a parent. You'll be creating memories that will last your children's lifetime! Just think—when you're seventy, your grown child will recollect at your big birthday bash all about how you put so much effort and creativity into those special themed meals . . .

Apply the Good Kind of Peer Pressure

If a child's admired friend always eats his vegetables, make sure to have him to dinner and point out how strong and smart and energetic that friend must be from eating all that healthy food.

Always Praise and Encourage Your Child . . .

Even if she only eats one or two mouthfuls of a super-healthy food, lavish her with praise and encouragement. If she refuses, don't make any fuss about it at all. Surely, you've heard that saying about catching more flies with honey than with vinegar. Make a big deal about success, but don't pour your energy into the behaviors you don't wish to encourage.

As you apply my advice, you'll find yourself coming up with your own personal variations on the themes of great diet and exercise, and I hope you'll share your expertise with friends to spread the *Family Fun and Fitness* word far and wide. You're on your way to being a fit family! I hope you've found these workouts and tips helpful, and I hope they can provide you with a foundation that will promote your family's best health now and in the years to come.

Fit Family Recipes

BREAKFAST IDEAS

HEARTY BREAKFAST OMELET

Serve for a hearty breakfast, or for lunch or dinner with a side order of vegetables.

YIELD: 4–5 SERVINGS

4 precooked, nitrate-free chicken or turkey sausages

1 teaspoon butter

2 teaspoons olive oil

2 cups of assorted vegetables

6 eggs

1 tablespoon water (very cold)

Salt and pepper

Spray oil

Sliced avocado (optional)

Small amount of grated flavorful cheese (optional)

Cut the chicken or sausage into bite-sized pieces and set them aside in a small bowl. Melt the butter with the oil in a medium-sized skillet with a heatproof handle, and cook the vegetables until crisp-tender, about 2 minutes. Spoon the vegetables out of the pan into the small bowl with the chicken or sausage pieces; stir to combine.

Beat the eggs well. Lightly season the eggs with salt and pepper, and add the water. Coat the pan with spray oil and heat the pan until very hot. Pour half the egg mixture into the pan. Holding the handle in one hand and a spatula in the other, push the egg mixture away from the edge of the pan, then tilt the pan to allow the uncooked egg to fill the open space on the pan's surface. Repeat until all the egg is cooked.

Add half the vegetable/meat mixture to one side of the pan. Add the avocado and/or cheese, if using. Flip the far edge of the egg over the mixture. Slide it out of the pan onto a plate, and repeat with the other half of the egg mixture and the veggie/meat mixture. Half this omelet is probably enough to serve an adult!

Tip: For vegetables, try cherry tomatoes, grated or chopped zucchini, scallions, spinach, diced onion, or others.

PEACH MELBA SMOOTHIE

This delicious smoothie is a cool treat on a hot day. You can turn it into a dessert shake by using ice cream instead of yogurt.

YIELD: 4–6 SERVINGS

4 frozen peaches or nectarines, peeled, pitted, and coarsely chopped (about 3 cups)

1 1/2 cups frozen raspberries

2 1/2 cups milk (dairy, soy, almond, or rice milk)

2 cups vanilla yogurt (or 4 decent scoops of good-quality vanilla ice cream)

Put all the ingredients into a blender or food processor, and process until smooth and creamy.

APPLE PECAN OATMEAL

Serve oatmeal with "spoonable" toppings.
You might be able to convince your kids that
this is like a sundae bar for breakfast!

SERVES 4–6

Oatmeal

1 1/2 cups slow-cooking rolled oats

3 cups water

Toppings

1 tart apple, chopped

1/4 cup raisins

1/4 cup crushed pecans or other nuts

1/2 cup plain or vanilla yogurt

2 tablespoons granola, or 1 tablespoon ground flaxseed plus
1 tablespoon flaked sweetened coconut (optional)

Maple syrup, agave syrup, or honey to taste

Cook oats in water according to package directions. Place the oatmeal in bowls and serve with bowls of apple, raisins, nuts, yogurt, other toppings, and sweetener, and let the kids doctor up their own oatmeal.

Expand your breakfast horizons. Consider other recipes in this section that would make a hearty and nutritious breakfast for you and your children: the Mini-Me Burger on page 172, for example, or the Potato and Bacon Frittata on page 174.

LUNCH AND DINNER IDEAS

MINESTRONE SOUP

*This soup takes some time, but is delicious—
and it makes for great leftovers.*

SERVES 4

1 tablespoon olive oil

1 onion, peeled and chopped

1 to 2 cloves garlic, crushed

1 large carrot, peeled and diced

5 cups vegetable stock

6 fresh ripe or one 8-ounce can of tomatoes, chopped

1 large potato, peeled and diced

$1/2$ can cannellini beans

$1/2$ cup peas

$1 1/2$ cups chopped cabbage

1 cup green beans, chopped

1 medium zucchini, chopped

2 tablespoons chopped parsley

2 tablespoons store-bought pesto

Salt and pepper

$1/2$ cup small pasta shapes

Freshly grated Parmesan cheese, to serve (optional)

Warm the oil in a soup pot. Add the onion and garlic and sauté for 10 minutes, or until the onion and garlic are golden brown. Add the carrots and continue to sauté for 2 more minutes. Add the stock, tomatoes, potato, cannellini beans, and peas. Bring to a boil; then reduce heat, and half cover the pan with a lid. Simmer for 40 minutes. Add the cabbage, green beans, zucchini, parsley, pesto, and salt and pepper to taste. Simmer for an additional 20 minutes. Add pasta and cook an additional 10 minutes, or until all the vegetables and pasta are soft. Grate Parmesan cheese over each bowl of soup just before serving.

BROCCOLI SALAD

A favorite salad for potlucks and cookouts.

YIELD: 6–8 SERVINGS

5 to 6 cups broccoli florets, broken into small pieces

6 slices good-quality bacon, crisply cooked

1/2 cup chopped red onion

3/4 cup mayonnaise

2 tablespoons sugar, honey, or agave nectar

2 tablespoons apple cider vinegar

Combine the broccoli florets, cooked bacon, and red onion in a medium-sized bowl. Mix the mayonnaise, sweetener, and vinegar together and toss with the other ingredients. Refrigerate one hour before serving to allow flavors to meld.

SAUSAGE PINEAPPLE RICE

Savory and sweet.

YIELD: 4–5 SERVINGS

*1/3 cup long-grain rice, rinsed
(brown rice, if your children will eat it)*

1 cup water

*8 ounces precooked, nitrate-free chicken
or turkey sausage*

2 tablespoons unsalted butter

Olive oil, for glazing

*3 tablespoons canned corn kernels,
drained and rinsed*

Generous 1/2 cup fresh pineapple, cubed

1 tablespoon finely chopped fresh parsley

Place the rice in a pan. Cover with the water and bring to a boil. Reduce heat, cover, and simmer for 15 minutes, or until the water has been absorbed and the rice is cooked. (Allow up to 45 minutes of cooking time if using brown rice.)

Cut the chicken or sausage into bite-sized pieces and set aside. Melt the butter in a small, heavy-bottomed pan. Add the corn and pineapple, and heat through for a minute or so. Add the rice, chicken or sausage, and parsley to the pan and stir well to combine.

CHICKEN AND APPLE BITES

A tasty combination of chicken and apple, mixed with whole-wheat bread crumbs. Make the bites small enough for finger food, or cut them up into bite-sized pieces.

YIELD: 4–5 SERVINGS

1 apple, peeled, cored, and grated

2 skinless, boneless, chicken breasts, cut into chunks

½ red onion, chopped

1 tablespoon chopped fresh parsley

Scant 1 cup fresh whole-wheat bread crumbs

1 tablespoon concentrated chicken stock

Whole-wheat flour, for coating

Canola, peanut, light olive, or sunflower seed oil, for pan-frying

Spread the grated apple out on a clean dish towel or paper towel and press out all the excess moisture.

Put the apple, chicken, onion, parsley, bread crumbs, and stock in a food processor and pulse briefly until well combined.

Spread the flour out on a plate. Divide the mixture into twenty or more mini-portions, shape each portion into a ball, and roll in the flour.

Heat a little oil in a large nonstick skillet over medium heat and cook the balls for 5 to 8 minutes, or until golden brown all over and cooked through. Remove and drain on paper towels. Serve hot or cold.

(Adapted from Sandra Baddeley's *Wholesome Meals for Babies and Toddlers*, Parragon Publishing, 2006)

SALMON FISH CAKES

We use fresh salmon to make these fish cakes, but canned salmon speeds up their preparation slightly.

YIELD: 8 CAKES

12 ounces salmon fillets, skinned and boned

Milk or water, for poaching

1 1/2 pounds potatoes, peeled and cut into chunks

1 tablespoon ketchup

2 teaspoons Dijon mustard

2 scallions, finely sliced

All-purpose flour, for dusting

Light olive, canola, or sunflower seed oil

Salt and pepper

Put the salmon in a large, shallow skillet and just cover with milk. Bring to a boil, then reduce the heat and let simmer for 3 to 4 minutes, or until just cooked. Lift the fish from the pan and reserve the poaching milk. Once the salmon has cooled, flake into large chunks and remove any stray bones.

Boil the potatoes in a large pan of water for 15 minutes, or until tender. Drain, return to pan, and mash with 2 to 3 tablespoons of the reserved poaching milk. The potatoes should be dry and smoothly mashed—no lumps.

Stir the ketchup, mustard, scallions, and half the salmon into the mashed potatoes. Season to taste with salt and pepper. Mix until well combined. Add the rest of the salmon to the potato mixture, mixing gently to avoid breaking up the fish pieces.

Dust a large plate (and your hands) with flour and shape the mixture into eight cakes. Lightly coat each cake in the flour, then put the cakes on a cookie sheet and cover with plastic wrap. Refrigerate for 30 minutes to firm up the cakes.

Generously coat the bottom of a large skillet with oil. Cook the fish cakes for 3 minutes on each side, or until crisp and golden. Keep the cooked fish cakes warm while cooking the remainder. Cut up into small pieces or mash for your child, depending on his age.

PENNE WITH CHICKEN AND PEAS

This simple dish always goes down well. Boost its nutrient content further by serving it with steamed broccoli. Try different pastas— such as those made with rice instead of wheat—for variety.

YIELD: 4–5 SERVINGS

10 ounces dried penne (rice, wheat, or other)

2 tablespoons olive oil

Two boneless, skinless chicken breasts or turkey cutlets

1 onion, very finely chopped

1 teaspoon dried oregano

2 garlic cloves, very finely chopped

Generous 1 cup vegetable or chicken stock

1¼ cups frozen baby peas

3 tablespoons sour cream, plus 3 tablespoons plain yogurt

Pepper (optional)

Freshly grated Parmesan cheese, to serve

Cook the pasta in a large pan of salted, boiling water according to the package directions. Drain, reserving 2 tablespoons of the cooking water.

Meanwhile, heat 2 tablespoons oil in a heavy-bottomed skillet. Salt and pepper the chicken breasts or turkey cutlets, and cook until a meat thermometer reads 160 to 165°F—about 4 to 5 minutes per side. (Pounding the breasts thin between two sheets of wax paper or inside a Ziploc bag will make for faster cooking. You don't need to do this with turkey cutlets.) Or you can use a countertop grill such as the George Foreman Grill to cook the chicken or turkey. Remove from heat quickly as soon as breasts/cutlets are cooked; when cool, cut into bite-sized chunks.

Add the onion to the pan (adding more oil if needed) and cook, stirring occasionally, for 8 minutes or until soft and slightly golden. Add the oregano and garlic and cook, stirring for 1 minute. Add the stock and bring to a boil, then reduce the heat and let simmer for 2 minutes.

Stir in the baby peas, chicken or turkey chunks, and the sour cream and yogurt. Cook over low heat, stirring frequently, until warmed through. Stir in the pasta and the reserved cooking water, then season to taste with fresh ground pepper, if desired. Serve sprinkled with Parmesan cheese.

Asian Noodles with Peanut Sauce

Good hot or room temperature, for lunch or dinner. You can add chunks of cooked boneless chicken, steak, or baked tofu to this dish.

YIELD: 4–5 SERVINGS

½ pound whole-wheat spaghetti

¼ cup soy sauce or tamari

2 tablespoons rice vinegar

1 tablespoon sesame oil

1 teaspoon hot sauce
(optional—use only if everyone likes a little spice!)

¼ cup natural peanut butter

1 cup sugar snap peas or shelled edamame
(green soybeans)

2 cups shredded cabbage (napa or other Asian cabbage will work,
or just use a bag of coleslaw mix)

Small amount of sliced red pepper (optional—adds color)

3 scallions, thinly sliced

2 tablespoons sesame seeds

Boil a pot of salted water to cook the spaghetti until *al dente* (slightly chewy)—about 9 minutes. Pour into colander, drain, rinse, and allow to drain completely.

Meanwhile, combine the soy sauce or tamari, rice vinegar, sesame oil, and hot sauce in a large plastic bowl. Warm the peanut butter in a microwave 10 to 15 seconds before whisking into other ingredients. Slice the snap peas, if using. (If using edamame, prepare according to package directions; you can't eat the pods of edamame, so if you couldn't find shelled edamame, enlist the kids' help to pop the bright green beans out of their pods before adding to the vegetable mixture.)

Add the cabbage and other veggies, plus the noodles, to the sauce in the large bowl. Toss until all ingredients are coated with sauce. Lightly toast the sesame seeds in a dry skillet for only 1 minute or so; sprinkle over noodles before serving.

PORK AND APPLE PAN-FRY

Another sweet, savory entrée the kids will love.

YIELD: 4–5 SERVINGS

1 tablespoon all-purpose flour

15 ounces pork tenderloin,
trimmed and cut into bite-sized pieces

2 tablespoons olive oil

1 onion, very finely chopped

2 garlic cloves, chopped

1 tablespoon fresh rosemary, very finely chopped

1 large carrot, peeled and very finely chopped

2 dessert apples, peeled, cored, and chopped

Generous 1 cup vegetable stock

3 tablespoons sour cream

Salt and pepper

Put the flour in a small Ziploc bag and season with salt and pepper. Add the pork. Shake the bag to coat the pork in the seasoned flour. Turn the pork out onto a plate and shake off any excess flour.

Heat the oil in a large, heavy-bottomed skillet and cook the pork over medium-high heat, turning frequently, for 5 minutes or until sealed and browned all over. Add the onion and garlic to the pan and cook, stirring occasionally, until softened. Mix in the rosemary, carrot, and apples, then cook for 4 minutes or until the apples begin to break down.

Pour in the stock and bring to a boil, then reduce the heat and let simmer, partially covered, for 15 to 20 minutes or until reduced and thickened. Stir in the sour cream and heat through before serving.

(Adapted from Sandra Baddeley's *Wholesome Meals for Babies and Toddlers*, Parragon Publishing, 2006)

SALMON AND BROCCOLI PASTA

A one-two nutritional punch: broccoli, full of antioxidant nutrition and fiber, and salmon, rich in healthy fats and protein— with a creamy, flavorful cream cheese kick.

YIELD: 4–5 SERVINGS

3 ounces dried small pasta shells (rice, wheat, or other)

$1/2$ cup broccoli florets

1 teaspoon unsalted butter

1 teaspoon olive oil

1 small onion, very finely chopped

5 ounces wild salmon fillet, skinned, boned, and cubed

4 tablespoons garlic/herb or plain cream cheese

2 to 3 tablespoons whole milk

Salt and pepper

Cook the pasta in a pot of salted, boiling water according to the package directions, then drain. Steam the broccoli for 7 to 10 minutes, or until tender.

Meanwhile, prepare the sauce. Melt the butter with the oil in a small, heavy-bottomed skillet and cook the onion, stirring occasionally, for 8 minutes or until softened. Add the salmon and cook for 2 minutes, or until just cooked and opaque. Stir in the cream cheese and milk, and heat through. Combine the sauce with the pasta and broccoli. Season with salt and freshly ground pepper.

MINI-ME BURGERS

*Kids love bite-sized foods—and these mini-burgers are
no exception! Skip the fries or chips and serve with
crisp, fresh vegetable sticks and Ranch dressing,
or with corn on the cob when it's in season.*

YIELD: 4–5 SERVINGS

Burger

$3/4$ cup fresh whole-wheat bread crumbs

Scant 2 cups fresh, lean ground beef,
ground chicken, or ground turkey

1 tablespoon tomato paste

1 egg, beaten

1 teaspoon dried oregano

1 onion, grated

1 carrot, peeled and grated

1 garlic clove, crushed

Vegetable oil, for pan-frying

Toppings

Mini-burger buns

Tomato slices

Lettuce leaves

Ketchup or relish of choice

Salt and pepper

Put all the burger ingredients, except the oil, in a large bowl and mix together with your hands until combined. Shape the mixture into balls. Cover with plastic wrap and refrigerate for 15 minutes.

Heat enough oil to cover the bottom of a large, heavy-bottomed skillet. Cook the burgers for 3 to 5 minutes, turning until browned all over. (Or use a countertop grilling machine.) Salt and pepper to taste. Serve each burger in a mini-burger bun with your kids' favorite toppings.

TASTY TACOS

These are great for getting you through those nights when you don't have a healthy dinner planned, but know you don't want to revert to dashing out for a fast-food feast!

YIELD: 4–5 SERVINGS

Corn tortillas

Spray oil

Leftover meat, chicken, or fish (optional) or ground turkey

1 16-ounce can black beans or pinto beans, drained and rinsed

Shredded or julienned cabbage or lettuce

Shredded cheddar or Monterey jack cheese

Plain yogurt

Mild salsa (optional)

Avocado or guacamole (optional, see page 175 for recipe)

Sliced black olives (optional)

Combine the beans and the meat and heat. Coat a small skillet with spray oil and warm the tortillas. Serve the ingredients in separate bowls so that kids can create their own tacos, piling the bean and meat mixture in with the other ingredients. Make sure you have plenty of napkins on hand!

Tip: Try the kind of beans that are pre-seasoned for Mexican dishes.

BACON AND POTATO FRITTATA

This frittata is similar to the Spanish tortilla.
It makes a great breakfast, too!

YIELD: 4–5 SERVINGS

2 to 3 slices good-quality bacon

1½ tablespoons olive oil

1 onion, very finely chopped

12 ounces new potatoes, cooked, and halved or quartered, if large

½ cup fast-cooking vegetable(s) of your choice

6 eggs, lightly beaten

Salt and pepper

Tomato wedges, to serve

Guacamole (optional, for recipe see page 175)

Spicy salsa (optional)

Preheat the broiler to high. Cook the bacon under the broiler until crisp. Let cool slightly, then chop into small pieces and set aside.

Heat the oil in a large, heavy-bottomed skillet with a heatproof handle, and cook the onion and other vegetables (reserving the potato), stirring occasionally, for 8 minutes or until softened. Add the potatoes and cook, turning frequently to prevent them sticking to the skillet, for 5 minutes or until golden.

Add the chopped bacon, then spread the veggie/bacon mixture evenly over the bottom of the skillet. Reheat the broiler to high. Beat the eggs in a medium-sized bowl. Lightly season the eggs with salt and fresh ground pepper, then pour carefully over the veggie/bacon mixture. Cook over medium heat for 5 to 6 minutes without disturbing, until the eggs are just set and the base of the frittata is lightly golden brown. Place the skillet under the broiler and cook the top for 3 minutes, until lightly golden.

Serve the frittata warm or cold, cut into wedges or slices, with fresh tomato wedges. Adults might enjoy some spicy salsa or guacamole with this dish.

Tip: For vegetables, try frozen baby peas, chopped spinach or other leafy greens, finely chopped red pepper, or grated zucchini with excess liquid squeezed out, or a combination.

CHICKEN FAJITAS WITH GUACAMOLE

A fun, festive, well-balanced and simple meal.

YIELD: 4–6 SERVINGS

Fajitas
1 teaspoon ground cumin
1 tablespoon olive oil, plus extra for brushing
1 garlic clove, sliced
Juice of 1 lime
4 chicken breasts, about 4 ounces each, cut into strips
Salt and pepper, to taste

Guacamole
1 large avocado, pitted, flesh scooped out and set aside
1 garlic clove, minced
Juice of 1/2 lemon
Salt and pepper, to taste

Tortillas
4 soft flour or corn tortillas
1 red bell pepper, seeded and sliced
1 scallion, finely sliced

Mix the cumin, oil, garlic, and lime juice together in a nonmetallic, shallow dish. Season the chicken with salt and pepper, then add to the dish and turn to coat in the marinade. Cover with plastic wrap. Let marinate in the refrigerator for up to 1 hour, turning occasionally.

To make the guacamole, mash the avocado, garlic, and lemon juice together in a bowl with a fork. Add the salt and pepper to taste and mix until smooth and creamy. Set aside.

Preheat a stovetop grill pan. Remove the chicken from the marinade and brush with oil, then cook for 6 to 8 minutes, turning halfway through the cooking time, until cooked through and golden.

Meanwhile, warm the tortillas. To serve in a kid-friendly way, arrange an equal quantity of the chicken, red bell pepper, and scallions down the center of each tortilla, add a spoonful of guacamole, and roll up; then, slice diagonally in half to serve.

HONEY SALMON KABOBS

The marinade in this recipe gives a wonderful, sweet, caramel flavor and glossy coating to the fish. While kabobs are fun, do take care when giving them to children. If you use wooden skewers, soak them in water first to prevent them from burning. You can substitute firm white fish, beef, pork, or chicken for the salmon in this recipe.

YIELD: 4–6 SERVINGS

Fish

4 boneless salmon fillets (about 5 ounces each), skinned and cut into $3/_4$-inch cubes

Marinade

2 tablespoons honey

2 tablespoons soy sauce

1 tablespoon olive oil

1 teaspoon toasted sesame oil

Accompaniments

Freshly cooked rice and peas, to serve

1 tablespoon toasted sesame seeds (optional)

Mix the marinade ingredients together in a shallow dish. Add the salmon and stir to coat in the marinade. Cover with plastic wrap and let marinate in the refrigerator for 1 hour, turning the fish occasionally.

Preheat the broiler to high and line the broiler pan with foil. Thread the cubes of salmon onto 4 to 6 skewers. Arrange on the broiler rack and brush with the marinade. Cook under the broiler for 3 to 5 minutes, turning frequently, until cooked through. Meanwhile, put the remaining marinade in a small pan and heat for a few minutes until it has reduced and thickened.

Serve the kabobs on a bed of rice and peas. Spoon the reduced marinade over the kabobs and sprinkle with the sesame seeds, if using.

CHILI FOR A CROWD

Having a party? Or looking for a meal that can be frozen in portions to heat up when dinner preparation is the last thing on your long list of to-dos? Look no further!

YIELD: 35–40 PORTIONS

Chili

$1/2$ cup good-quality olive oil

$13/4$ pounds yellow onions, coarsely chopped

5 pounds sweet Italian sausage with casings removed
or 5 pounds homemade Italian turkey sausage
(see next page for recipe)

$11/2$ tablespoons ground fresh pepper

24 ounces tomato paste

3 tablespoons minced garlic

6 tablespoons ground cumin

8 tablespoons chili powder

$1/2$ cup Dijon mustard

4 tablespoons salt

4 tablespoons dried basil

4 tablespoons dried oregano

6 pounds canned Italian plum tomatoes,
drained and chopped

$1/2$ cup red wine

$1/4$ cup fresh lemon juice

$1/2$ cup chopped fresh dill

$1/2$ cup chopped fresh Italian parsley

3 16-ounce cans dark red kidney beans or black beans,
drained and rinsed

Homemade Italian Turkey Sausage

5 pounds lean ground turkey

10 teaspoons garlic powder

7½ teaspoons crushed fennel seed

7½ teaspoons sugar

5 teaspoons salt

5 teaspoons dried oregano

2½ teaspoons dried pepper

Heat the olive oil in a very large heavy pot. Add the onions and cook over low heat, covered, until tender about 10 minutes. Crumble the sausage meat into the pot and cook over medium-high heat, stirring often, until meat is well browned.

Turn the heat to medium-low and stir in the black pepper, tomato paste, garlic, cumin, chili powder, mustard, salt, basil, and oregano. Add the drained tomatoes, wine, lemon juice, dill, parsley, and kidney or black beans. Stir well and simmer, uncovered, for another 20 minutes. Taste and correct the seasoning. Once heated through, serve immediately.

Tip: If using homemade Italian turkey sausage, it will need to be prepared the night before you cook with it. In a large bowl, combine ground turkey with garlic powder, fennel seed, sugar, salt, oregano, and pepper. Cover with plastic wrap and refrigerate overnight. Use in place of store-bought Italian sausage in any recipe.

Pasta with Sausage and Sautéed Spinach

*Another recipe where you can
use the homemade sausage!*

YIELD: 4–6 SERVINGS

1 16-ounce package of whole-wheat blend
thin spaghetti or other pasta

2 tablespoons olive oil

1 pound sweet Italian sausage with casings removed
or 1 pound turkey or chicken sausage

2 cloves garlic, minced

2 1/2 cups chicken broth

1/8 teaspoon red pepper flakes

1 package fresh baby spinach

4 tablespoons unsalted butter

1 1/2 cups Parmesan cheese

1 teaspoon salt

1 teaspoon fresh ground pepper

Cook the pasta according to package directions. Meanwhile, in a large saucepan, over medium heat, heat the oil. Add the sausage and cook, crumbling it with a spoon, until browned, about 5 minutes. Add the garlic and cook for 1 minute more.

Add the broth and red pepper and bring to a boil. Then add the spinach, cover, and cook until tender—about 3 minutes. Stir in the butter and Parmesan cheese and cook, uncovered, until the sauce thickens slightly, about 2 minutes. Add the drained pasta, season with salt and pepper, and toss to combine.

Tasty . . . our kids love it. Great for leftovers!

DESSERT IDEAS

OATMEAL-CHOCOLATE CHIP COOKIES

This great cookie recipe is based on one from a book by Cynthia Lair called Feeding the Whole Family: Whole Foods Recipes for Babies, Young Children and Their Parents *(Moon Smile Press, Seattle, WA, 1994). They're fun to make with children—the batter is rolled by hand and gently squooshed onto the baking sheet. They have a taste like a slightly sweet granola bar.*

YIELD: ABOUT 20 COOKIES

$1\frac{1}{2}$ cup slow-cooking rolled oats

1 cup all-purpose flour

$\frac{1}{4}$ teaspoon salt

$\frac{1}{2}$ cup maple syrup

$\frac{1}{3}$ melted butter or cold-pressed vegetable oil

1 teaspoon vanilla

$\frac{1}{3}$ cup chopped nuts, flaked unsweetened coconut, or dried cranberries (or a combination)

$\frac{1}{3}$ cup chocolate chips

Preheat oven to 350°F. Combine dry ingredients in a large bowl except for nuts and chocolate chips. Combine wet ingredients in a small bowl, then combine wet and dry ingredients, including the nuts and chocolate chips.

Moisten hands and form dough into balls big enough to make 3-inch cookies. Place on a lightly oiled baking sheet and gently press with palm into cookie shape. Bake 15 to 20 minutes, or until golden at edges.

Variation: Substitute $\frac{1}{2}$ cup of almond meal for $\frac{1}{2}$ cup of all-purpose flour if you can find it; this adds moistness and a lot of good nutrition.

YOGURT PARFAIT

A tasty, healthful, colorful dessert you can feel good about serving to your kids. It also works for breakfast!

YIELD: 4 SERVINGS

2 cups plain or vanilla yogurt
2 cups fresh or frozen fruit, cut into chunks, if necessary
2 cups low-fat granola
Gingersnap cookies, to serve (optional)

Place several spoonfuls of yogurt on the bottom of each sundae glass. Add fresh seasonal or frozen fruit and low-fat granola, and follow with another layer of yogurt. Top with a gingersnap cookie for a festive touch.

HEALTHY SUNDAE

This healthy twist on the classic ice-cream sundae is sure to become a firm favorite . . . fun to make with the kids on a hot weekend!

YIELD: SERVES 4

1 large mango, seeded, peeled, and coarsely chopped
1 tablespoon chopped mixed nuts or slivered almonds (optional)
4 scoops good-quality vanilla ice cream
Handful of chopped strawberries, to decorate
4 teddy-shaped cookies, to serve (optional)

Put the mango flesh in a blender or food processor and process until blended and smooth. Press through a strainer to remove any fibers from the mango.

Lightly toast the nuts, if using, in a dry skillet. Let cool.

To serve, place a few spoonfuls of the mango purée in each of four sundae glasses. Top with a scoop of ice cream. Spoon over more of the mango purée. Decorate with the strawberries and nuts, and serve with the cookies, if using.

Variation: Instead of mango, try strawberry, peach, or nectarine purée.

SMOOTHIE POPS

Use homemade smoothie to make healthy popsicles—
a great summertime treat.

YIELD: Depends on the size
of the paper cup or mold

2 cups frozen fruit (mango, strawberries,
and blueberries are especially good)

2/3 cup plain yogurt

Enough fruit juice (apple, papaya, orange,
pineapple, or other sweet or citrus juices will work)
to make a smoothie-like texture when blended

Blend together ingredients in a blender or food processor, and process until smooth and creamy. Pour the mixture into paper cups; cover with plastic wrap and insert a Popsicle stick into the center of each cup. Freeze until firm. To eat, peel away the cup. You can also make these with a store-bought Popsicle mold.

You can make these a bit sweeter by adding some vanilla or strawberry ice cream to the blender while making your smoothies.

Tip: Take advantage of fruit in season by buying lots of it to freeze. Place the fruit on a cookie tray when you first put it in the freezer; then, when it's partially frozen, you can pour it into a Ziploc bag. This prevents the pieces of fruit from sticking together. Some kids love to munch on frozen fruit when it's hot outside!

MELON FRUIT BOWL

If your child needs extra encouragement to eat fruit, then this attractive fruit-filled melon is bound to appeal. Make the fruit salad just before serving to retain as much of the fruits' nutrients as possible. This one's great for breakfast, too!

YIELD: 3–4 SERVINGS

1/2 large melon, seeded

A selection of fresh fruit

2 tablespoons fresh orange juice

Cut a sliver off the base of the melon half so that it stands upright, and place on a serving plate. Scoop out most of the flesh using a melon baller or teaspoon to leave a hollow bowl shape. Put the melon balls and the remaining fruit in a large bowl and pour over the orange juice. Turn to coat the fruit in the juice, then spoon the fruit into the melon shell. Pour over any remaining juice.

Tip: Choose fruits that are in seasons and popular, such as strawberries, raspberries, blueberries, orange segments, seedless grapes, slices of peach or nectarine, and chunks of banana.

GRILLED OR BROILED FRUIT KABOBS

Kids love to help make these kabobs before they go on the grill or under the broiler. If using wooden skewers, soak in water for 10 minutes before using.

YIELD: 4–6 SERVINGS

4 cups mixed cut fruit, such as mango, pineapple, banana, and strawberry

4 tablespoons butter, melted

2 tablespoons fresh lime juice

1 tablespoon honey (optional)

Skewers

Grill pan or basket (if grilling outdoors)

Vanilla ice cream or yogurt (optional)

If grilling: While preheating the grill, cut the fruit into $1\frac{1}{2}$-inch pieces. Place on skewers. Combine the butter, lime juice, and honey if using, and brush fruit with mixture. Place into grill pan or basket at least 2 inches from coals, making sure to prevent the fruit from catching fire. Grill for 5 minutes per side.

If broiling: Preheat the broiler while cutting the fruit and putting on skewers. Place the fruit on baking sheet and brush with the butter/lime juice/honey mixture. Broil for $1\frac{1}{2}$ minutes, about 5 inches from heat. Turn the skewers, brush again, and broil $1\frac{1}{2}$ minutes more.

This fruit is delicious with ice cream or dipped in plain or vanilla yogurt!

Variation: You can also serve fresh fruit on skewers. Try combinations of fresh melon, strawberries, pineapple, mango, and banana.

More Family Fun and Fitness to Come

For additional resources and ideas for keeping the whole family excited about being healthy, active, and fit, go to

www.fitnessforfamilyfun.com

There you'll find:

- More parent/child workouts

- More recipes for wholesome, healthy meals

- More ideas for enriching family traditions

- More examples of fit family teachable moments

- More valuable MVP Dad and Mom principles

- More research showing how fitness and nutrition promote optimal social and mental well-being, physical health, and academic achievement

- More tips and tricks to keep your new healthy family lifestyle challenging and fun in the long run

Index

About the Author

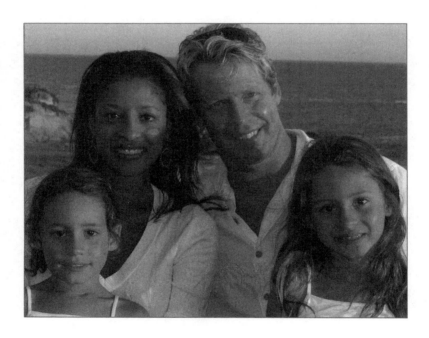

Knute Keeling grew up in Texas and Oklahoma. Playing sports in high school and college sparked his early interest in health and fitness, inspiring him to learn more in order to become a stronger and faster athlete. A near-fatal motorcycle accident put his athletic career on hold, but it led him to his current passion: fitness training and sports therapy.

While managing multi-million-dollar fitness facilities for Bally's in Southern California, Keeling fulfilled his dream of becoming a certified fitness specialist. He left the corporate health club world to start his own private training business at Laguna Health Club in Laguna Beach, California. His training business encompasses general health, disease prevention, and rehabilitation therapy, as well as training for athletes of all age groups and skill levels—youth, college, and professional. Keeling has been recognized as one of Southern California's top trainers by *Orange Coast Magazine*.

The author also delivers corporate health and wellness lectures designed to give employees tools for staying fit and healthy, even when traveling. He can be found most mornings and afternoons at the Laguna Health Club with his wonderful clients. However, he considers this to be his second job; his first and favorite job is that of an involved and passionate parent. He has been married for nine wonderful years to his wife, Nikki; they have two beautiful daughters, Cameron (age eight) and Kianna (age six).